The Supermarket Guide

Food Choices for You and Your Family

Written for
The American Dietetic Association
by Mary Abbott Hess
LHD, MS, RD, FADA

JOHN WILEY & SONS, INC.

New York • Chichester • Weinheim • Brisbane • Singapore • Toronto

The Supermarket Guide

Food Choices for You and Your Family

Written for The American Dietetic Association by
Mary Abbott Hess, LHD, MS, RD, FADA
assisted by Jane Grant Tougas

The American Dietetic Association Reviewers:
Heather Earls, RD
American Heart Association
Chicago, Illinois

Shari Steinback, MS, RD
Spartan Stores
Grand Rapids, Michigan

Susan Sundram, MS, RD
Shaw's Supermarket, Inc.
East Bridgewater, Massachusetts

Technical Editor:
Raeanne Sutz Sarazen, RD
The American Dietetic Association
Chicago, Illinois

THE AMERICAN DIETETIC ASSOCIATION is the largest group of food and health professionals in the world. As the advocate of the profession, the ADA serves the public by promoting optimal nutrition, health, and well-being.

For expert answers to your nutrition questions, call the ADA/ National Center for Nutrition and Dietetics Hot Line at (900) 225-5267. To listen to recorded messages or obtain a referral to a registered dietitian (RD) in your area, call (800) 366-1655. Visit the ADA's Website at www.eatright.org.

Contents

Bread, Cereal, Rice, and Pasta—31 *Breads and Bread Products; Baking Mixes; Cereal, Pasta, Rice, and Grains; Crackers; Cookies, Bars, and Snack Cakes; Packaged Snack Foods*

Vegetables—43 *Fresh, Frozen, Canned and Bottled*

Fruits—52 *Fresh, Frozen, Canned and Bottled, Dried*

Milk, Yogurt, and Cheese—61 *Milk and Milk Alternatives, Yogurt and Yogurt Products, Cheese and Cheese Products, Puddings and Custards*

Meat, Poultry, Fish, Dry Beans, Eggs, and Nuts—69 *Beef, Pork, Lamb, Veal, and Game Meats; Poultry and Game Birds; Fish and Seafood; Packaged Meats/Cold Cuts; Legumes; Eggs and Egg Substitutes; Nuts and Seeds/Nut Butters*

Fats, Oils, and Sweets—84 *Butter, Margarine, and Spreads; Cooking Fats; Vegetable Oils; Salad Dressings; Cream and Cream Substitutes; Frozen Desserts; Sugars, Syrups, Sweet Sauces, and Toppings; Jellies and Fruit Spreads*

Combined Foods—95 *Soups, Sauces, and Dips; Prepared Entrées; Baked Desserts; Deli Choices and Carry-Out Foods*

Beverages—100 *Coffee, Tea, and Cocoa; Soft Drinks, Sports Drinks, Water, and Flavored Waters; Wine, Beer, and Liquor*

Seasonings and Condiments—104

Baking Basics—105

Chapter One
Healthy Foods, Healthy Eating

IT'S NO SECRET that health and well-being are influenced by the choices we make in life. Even common, everyday choices have an impact. Take the food you eat, for instance. Over time, healthy eating habits can promote excellent health. They can also help you boost resistance to illness.

Making healthy food choices is what this book is all about. Use it as an aisle-by-aisle supermarket guide to making informed decisions about the food you buy for yourself and your family.

As you know, there's no shortage of choices to be made at the supermarket. Is corn on your shopping list? Should it be fresh, frozen, or canned? How about cereal? Should you go with a granola type or is presweetened OK?

And then there's the sometimes confusing nutrition and ingredient information on labels. What exactly does it mean and how should it influence your shopping decisions? Not to be forgotten is the important element of food prices. Is a whole chicken a better buy than precut pieces even if you have to discard bones and other parts?

This handy book provides the answers to these and hundreds more questions.

You will start by learning how to quickly use the nutrition and ingredient labels as you shop, as well as evaluate health claims touted on packaging. To make shopping an even more rewarding experience, you'll receive tips on getting more for your food dollar.

Then, in Chapter 4, we'll take a close look at specific foods organized by food groups. Not only will you find out which foods give you the biggest nutrition bang for your buck—those that are nutrient-rich but moderate in calories, fat, sugar, and salt—but you'll probably find many new food options to look for and try. And the "Shoppers Should Know" sections will provide new and interesting facts to make you a more discerning shopper: how foods in each group compare to each other, current nutrition information, and food safety and storage tips.

Finally, in Chapter 5, you'll find even more food safety recommendations.

Nutrition Guidelines

The advice provided within this book follows the recommendations of the Dietary Guidelines for Americans. These seven guidelines, which are the basis for nutrition policy in the United States, promote a healthful diet for people 2 years of age and older.

The Dietary Guidelines for Americans

1. Eat a variety of foods to get the energy, protein, vitamins, minerals, and fiber you need for good health.
2. Balance the food you eat with physical activity—maintain or improve your weight to reduce your chances of developing a problem associated with being overweight, such as high blood pressure, heart disease, a stroke, certain cancers, and adult-onset diabetes.
3. Choose a diet with plenty of grain products, vegetables, and fruits. These foods provide needed vitamins, minerals, fiber, and complex carbohydrates for good health and can help you lower your fat intake.
4. Choose a diet low in fat, saturated fat, and cholesterol to reduce your risk of heart disease and certain types of cancer. High levels of saturated fat and cholesterol in the diet are linked to increased blood cholesterol levels and obesity.
5. Choose a diet moderate in sugars. Some foods that contain a lot of sugar supply too many calories and too few

nutrients for most people and can contribute to tooth decay.

6. Choose a diet moderate in salt and sodium, which may help reduce your risk of high blood pressure.

7. If you drink alcoholic beverages, do so in moderation. Alcoholic beverages supply calories but little or no nutrients. Drinking alcohol is also the cause of many health problems and accidents and can lead to addiction.

The challenge is to translate this advice into realistic food choices. For instance, nearly everyone buys some high-calorie, high-sugar, and high-sodium foods because they are their favorites or because the occasion is special. Fortunately, there is room in a healthy diet for any favorite food—particularly if you eat moderate portions.

That necessary flexibility is reflected in the Food Guide Pyramid, which the federal government designed to ensure variety and the availability of nutrients essential to good health. The Pyramid (see next page) graphically groups together foods that provide similar nutrients and suggests the number of daily servings to eat from each group.

Every healthy person, age 2 and older, should follow the Pyramid's guidelines and eat more servings of foods from the base of the Pyramid (grain products, vegetables, and fruits) and fewer servings of foods from the tip (sugars and fats). This will not only provide the nutrients that you and your family need but will help you to achieve or maintain a healthy weight.

Each food group contains a number of choices. Different foods within the same group provide varying amounts of fat, saturated fat, cholesterol, sugar, and sodium. For example, you can have your sandwich on a French bread roll that provides 1 gram of fat or on a croissant that provides 12 grams of fat. Both of these 2-ounce bread portions count as 2 servings from the grain group but have differing amounts of fat and calories.

Remember, all foods can fit into a healthy diet, but it takes knowledge and practice to learn which foods should be eaten most often and which foods should be chosen less frequently.

Eating should bring pleasure, comfort, and joy, and not create

Healthy Foods, Healthy Eating

feelings of deprivation or guilt. But do yourself a favor. Try to balance your "indulge me" favorites with plenty of foods listed in Chapter 4's "Look For" sections. That way, your entire market basket will provide you and your family with a total diet that promotes wonderful eating and good health.

The Food Guide Pyramid
A Guide to Healthy Choices

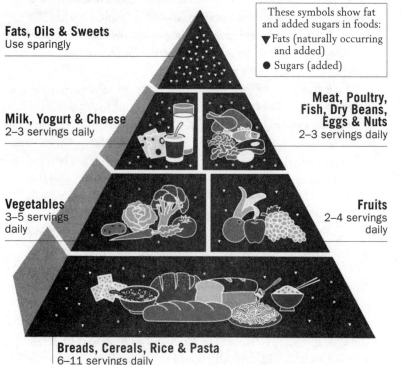

Fats, Oils & Sweets
Use sparingly

These symbols show fat and added sugars in foods:
▼ Fats (naturally occurring and added)
● Sugars (added)

Milk, Yogurt & Cheese
2–3 servings daily

Meat, Poultry, Fish, Dry Beans, Eggs & Nuts
2–3 servings daily

Vegetables
3–5 servings daily

Fruits
2–4 servings daily

Breads, Cereals, Rice & Pasta
6–11 servings daily

U.S. Department of Agriculture/U.S. Department of Health and Human Services, 1992.

Chapter Two
It's On the Label

SMART SHOPPERS TAKE FULL ADVANTAGE of the government-mandated labeling system that provides a wealth of nutrition information in a standard format. Everything from the Nutrition Facts panel to the ingredient list to the regulated descriptive terms on the front of the label will help you compare foods and make choices that better meet your health needs.

Although most foods sold in supermarkets provide nutrient and ingredient information right on the package, certain foods are exempt from labeling laws. These foods include fresh products, such as raw fruits, vegetables, seafood, poultry, and meat that would be difficult to label; products from very small manufacturers who may not be able to afford to label; and foods that provide little or no nutrients, such as coffee, tea, and water.

Although not required, many stores provide information on vegetables, fruits, meat, and seafood or on signs where the food is sold. And some manufacturers of bottled water, particularly fruit-flavored waters with no calories, choose to provide label information. Foods with small or unusual package sizes are permitted to use a modified label format. Foods for babies and children under 2 years of age use a different label format based on the nutrients young eaters need.

Manufacturers may list nutrients beyond the ones required and sometimes choose to do so, particularly if a food is an excellent source of a nutrient.

The Nutrition Facts Label

Using the Nutrition Facts food label is a key strategy for healthy eating. Directly under the label's "Nutrition Facts" title appears a serving size and the number of servings in the container. This information is important because the calories and nutrient data on the rest of the label relate to the specified portion size which may be as small as 1 teaspoon or as large as 1 cup.

When comparing food labels on similar items, first look to be sure that the portions are the same. For foods in single-serving containers, a portion is usually the whole container. For example, you may see 4-, 6-, and 8-ounce single-serving packages of yogurt as well as quart containers. However, if you compare labels for nutrients without realizing the differences in portion size, you will be misled. All the nonfat yogurts, for example, will probably have similar nutrient values for the same size portions.

It is also important to adjust the stated serving size to what you will actually eat. If the label says that a serving is 3 ounces of meat, and you will eat 6 ounces, expect to enjoy twice the calories and nutrients.

The next part of the label lists eight nutrients, their % Daily Values, and how much of each nutrient is in a serving. Total fat, cholesterol, sodium, total carbohydrate, dietary fiber, sugars, and protein are included.

Some nutrients listed on the label are probably more important to you than others, depending on your individual needs and health concerns. Most people are concerned about choosing a heart-healthy diet low in total fat and saturated fat. Unless your blood cholesterol is high, you may not need to pay much attention to the amount of cholesterol in the food you eat. Only about 10 percent of the general population experience elevated blood cholesterol levels from cholesterol found in food. Diets high in total fat, particularly saturated fats, are much more likely to raise your blood cholesterol level.

Sodium may be important to you if your blood pressure is elevated. People with diabetes must be aware of total carbohydrate intake, and vegetarians need to ensure adequate iron, calcium, and vitamin B12 intake. People with kidney problems usually

Nutrition Facts

Serving Size 1 cup (248g)
Servings Per Container 4

Amount Per Serving

Calories 150   Calories from Fat 35

	% Daily Value*
Total Fat 4g	**6%**
Saturated Fat 2.5g	**12%**
Cholesterol 20mg	**7%**
Sodium 170mg	**7%**
Total Carbohydrate 17g	**6%**
Dietary Fiber 0g	**0%**
Sugars 17g	
Protein 13g	

Vitamin A 4%	•	Vitamin C 6%
Calcium 40%	•	Iron 0%

* Percent Daily Values are based on a 2,000
calorie diet. Your daily values may be higher or
lower depending on your calorie needs:

		Calories:	2,000	2,500
Total Fat	Less than		65g	80g
Sat Fat	Less than		20g	25g
Cholesterol	Less than		300mg	300mg
Sodium	Less than		2,400mg	2,400mg
Total Carbohydrate			300g	375g
Dietary Fiber			25g	30g

Calories per gram:

Fat 9   •   Carbohydrate 4   •   Protein 4

need to restrict protein and sodium and monitor potassium intake.

The dietary fiber information appearing on the label is not used as often as it should be. Most Americans don't eat enough dietary fiber. Fiber helps you lower the risk of heart disease and certain cancers, and reduces constipation, while aiding in weight control. Most of us should be seeking more sources of dietary fiber from grains, vegetables, legumes, and whole fruits.

% Daily Value: What Does It Mean?

You can use the % Daily Value (DV) as a general guide to good sources of some nutrients, maintaining low intakes of others (such as fat and saturated fat), and comparing the nutrient levels of similar food. Selecting foods that are good or excellent sources of vitamins and minerals is wise unless you have a medical problem that benefits from restricting one of these nutrients.

Basically, 100 percent of the % Daily Value for each nutrient is an estimate of an appropriate daily amount of that nutrient to be obtained from a variety of foods in a 2,000-calorie daily diet. If a particular food provides 0 to 9 percent of the % Daily Value for a nutrient, it is not a good source of that nutrient. Good sources of nutrients fall between 10 and 19 percent of the Daily Value. But if it provides 20 percent or more of the % Daily Value, it is rich in that particular nutrient and an excellent source.

More is not always better, though. Try not to exceed the 100% Daily Value for fat, saturated fat, cholesterol, or sodium on most days. But try to seek greater percentages—at least 100 percent of the Daily Value—for fiber, vitamins, and minerals (except sodium) because these nutrients promote health and help prevent certain diseases.

The portion of the label listing vitamin A, vitamin C, calcium, and iron gives only percentages of the Daily Values and not the actual amount of these nutrients. Vitamins A and C build strong cell walls and promote resistance to infections; calcium and iron protect against osteoporosis and anemia, respectively.

Daily Value percentages on the Nutrition Facts food label are based on a 2,000-calorie daily intake, but you may need more or fewer calories to maintain a healthy weight. Adjusting daily calories will change percentages of some nutrients.

Few people, however, have the time or inclination to measure, record, and adjust food choices or amounts to ensure they reach 100 percent of the Daily Values. Even though specific percentages may not apply to your diet, you can still use % Daily Values to see which foods are sources of key nutrients. For example, if fat, cholesterol, or sodium is restricted in your diet, think twice about foods that provide more than 10 percent of the Daily Value of those substances in a single serving.

Label Battles

A few controversies about nutrition labels are still brewing. For example, the label breaks out saturated fat from the total fat numbers. At this time, manufacturers are not required to list amounts of other types of fat— monounsaturated or polyunsaturated fat—although manufacturers of some products high in monounsaturated fat voluntarily list this number.

Some advocates want the government to mandate including trans-fatty acids on the label and to count them as saturated fats. Recent data suggests that trans-fatty acids, a rearranged form of monounsaturated fat, may act like saturated fat in the body. But much research is still needed, and scientific consensus must be reached before this change is made. In the "Shoppers Should Know" sections of Chapter 4, foods with trans-fatty acids are identified for you.

You also may note that there is no % Daily Value listed for sugars, although grams of sugars are listed. Health authorities have not yet agreed on an appropriate Daily Value for sugars for the typical person. The grams of sugars listed on the label include a total of all sources of sugars—both naturally occurring and added. Fruits, some vegetables, and milk contain sugars as a natural part of their composition. Sucrose (table sugar), corn syrup (liquid sugar), or other forms of sugars may be added in food processing. As in homemade foods, manufacturers use various types and amounts of sugars in recipes to provide desired flavors and textures. Naturally occurring and added sugars are used exactly the same way in the body. Some people need to monitor total carbohydrate intake, which includes sugars, to control blood sugar fluctuations or weight.

The Ingredients of a Healthy Diet

Food manufacturers are required to list all ingredients by weight from the most to least. For example, if a canned soup has tomatoes as the first item on its ingredient list, that means the soup contains more tomatoes by weight than anything else. Ingredients found at the end of the list are present in the smallest amounts.

If you have food sensitivities or allergies you should carefully read the ingredient listing to avoid any ingredient that will result in a reaction. Specific questions about ingredients should be directed to the food manufacturer. Many manufacturers offer a toll-free number to answer questions about their products and ingredients.

Making Their Claims

It is hard to miss the food packages that tout special nutritional attributes, such as fat-free or sugar-free. These nutrient content claims, usually printed in big letters and bright colors, can help speed your shopping and expand your food horizons. Checking the front of the product label can help you find fat-free, light, low-fat, and low-calorie foods.

Remember that fresh fruits and vegetables, although not labeled with nutrient content claims, are naturally low in calories, cholesterol-free, and low-fat or fat-free. Some foods labeled low-fat or reduced-fat have other ingredients added that replace many of the calories from fat. For example, some reduced-calorie salad dressings have added sugar for flavor or carbohydrates as thickeners. So always check the Nutrition Facts panel for calories as well as fat.

Some common product label nutrient content claims and their meanings are:

Calorie-free: less than 5 calories per serving

Fat-free or sugar-free: less than 1/2 gram of fat or sugar per serving

Low-calorie: 40 calories or less per serving

Low-sodium: less than 140 milligrams of sodium per serving of most foods; and 140 milligrams or less sodium per 100 grams of complete meals such as frozen dinners

Low-cholesterol: 20 milligrams or less cholesterol and 2 grams or less saturated fat per serving

Reduced: altered to contain 25 percent less of the specified nutrient or calories than the usual product

Good source (of vitamins or minerals): provides 10 to 19 percent or more of Daily Value of that vitamin or mineral per serving

High in: provides 20 percent or more of the Daily Value of the specified nutrient per serving

High fiber: 5 or more grams of fiber per serving

Light foods are altered so that they contain 1/3 fewer calories or 1/2 of the fat of the usual food. A light food that has most of its calories from fat must reduce fat by at least half.

Foods labeled **healthy** are low in fat and saturated fat and have limited sodium and cholesterol. And most healthy foods must provide at least 10 percent of the Daily Value of vitamin A, vitamin C, iron, protein, calcium, or fiber. By law, all fresh fruits and vegetables, single or mixed canned and frozen fruits and vegetables, and some enriched cereal grain products may be called healthy even if they do not contain 10 percent of a key nutrient.

Lean meats, poultry, seafood, and game have less than 10 grams of fat, less than 4 1/2 grams of saturated fat and less than 95 milligrams of cholesterol per 3 1/2 ounce cooked serving.

Extra lean meats, poultry, seafood, and game have less than 5 grams of fat, less than 2 grams of saturated fat, and less than 95 milligrams of cholesterol per 3 1/2 ounce cooked serving.

Claims About Health

To help you identify foods that fit into particular diets, the government strictly regulates the health claims that can appear on the front label of packaged foods. Eleven areas in which health claims are currently allowed include:

1. A calcium-rich diet may help prevent osteoporosis (thin, fragile bones).
2. Limiting the amount of sodium you eat may help prevent hypertension (high blood pressure).
3. Limiting the amount of saturated fat and cholesterol you eat may help prevent heart disease.
4. Eating fruits, vegetables, and grain products that contain fiber may help prevent heart disease.
5. Limiting the amount of total fat you eat may help reduce your risk for some types of cancer.
6. Eating high-fiber grain products, fruits, and vegetables may help prevent some types of cancer.

7. Eating fruits and vegetables that are low in fat and good sources of dietary fiber, vitamin A, or vitamin C may help prevent some types of cancer.
8. Women eating adequate amounts of folate, a B vitamin, daily throughout their childbearing years may reduce their risk of having a child with a neural tube birth defect.
9. Eating soluble fiber from whole oats as part of a diet low in saturated fat and cholesterol may help prevent heart disease.
10. Foods containing soluble fiber from psyllium seed husk (certain breakfast cereals) as part of a diet low in saturated fat and cholesterol may reduce risk of coronary heart disease.
11. Eating foods with sugar alcohols does not promote tooth decay.

Other Label Information

Individuals who keep kosher look for one of several symbols on the label that indicate that the food has met particular content, sanitation, and processing standards of an authorized Jewish food inspector. This is entirely voluntary and done in addition to government safety inspection.

The kosher symbols, which appear on a variety of foods throughout the store, do not validate any nutritional qualities. Different certifying groups use these and other symbols.

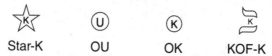

| Star-K | OU | OK | KOF-K |

A few foods carry health warnings for people with special health needs. Foods and beverages made with aspartame, a nonnutritive sweetener, carry warnings for people with phenylketonuria (PKU), a metabolic disease. Aspartame contains the essential amino acid phenylalanine, which can not be properly metabolized by people with PKU. Those with this disease must greatly restrict all protein-containing foods and have no need to use sugar substitutes anyway.

Some individuals are sensitive to sulfites, an additive used in food processing that preserves color and freshness. The words "contains sulfites" can be found on labels of some beer, wine, and dried fruits. Alcoholic beverages also carry warnings for pregnant women that drinking can result in birth defects.

The Truth, The Whole Truth

Remember that manufacturers frequently make changes in the foods they produce based on ingredient prices, preferred flavors, and sales data. By law, what is stated on the label (with small allowances for crop and seasonal differences), must be in the package. It's smart to check the labels on foods you buy frequently to be sure nothing has changed. The information in this book reflects food values of products on the market at press time.

Food manufacturers, especially major ones, are usually careful that the nutrient information on their labels is accurate. There are serious legal consequences for not meeting federal labeling requirements. Unfortunately, some manufacturers are not so careful and have been known to make unsubstantiated and untrue claims about their foods.

Deceptive labeling is not only unfair, it is dangerous for people with food allergies or those who must carefully monitor their intake of specific nutrients for medical reasons. Be especially cautious with foods sold in delis, bakeries, and health food stores, and keep in mind that if something tastes "too good to be true" the label information might be wrong.

If you are concerned about a specific food, talk to a dietitian about it or call the closest regional office of the Food and Drug Administration. FDA consumer affairs officers are excellent sources of information, and they are dedicated fraud-fighters.

Chapter Three

Stretching Your Food Dollar

MOST SHOPPERS FILL THEIR MARKET BASKETS with about 75 percent of the same products almost every week. Pay particular attention to economical choices when it comes to the foods you buy repeatedly. A look at your register receipts will tell you which foods to look at closely in terms of price and value. Learn to compare prices and become aware of how much you are paying for value-added convenience items. You can save money by relying on these three tools: a well-planned shopping list, coupons and rebates, and in-store sales.

The Shopping List

Efficient shoppers almost always use a list. Organize your shopping list by food categories, preferably in the aisle-by-aisle layout of the store. Start your shopping list at the first aisle as you enter the store. Develop a standard form that includes foods you typically buy in each category along with space to write down other items you wish to add. Some supermarkets offer printed shopping lists that you can customize to reflect your special needs.

Keep your shopping list handy at home so you can jot down staples you are running out of and fresh foods you have used and want to replace. To finish your list, decide what recipes you will be making in the week to come and what foods you will need.

Plan to use produce that keeps longer in the refrigerator (like broccoli, cabbage, carrots, grapefruit, and tangerines) later in the week and more perishable items like fresh corn, ripe peaches, or Boston lettuce earlier in the week when it is at its peak flavor and texture. If you are buying fruit to eat today or tomorrow, buy it ripe. If you will use it later in the week, buy it less ripe. For example, most stores have bananas ripe and ready-to-eat as well as firmer ones that will be tastier in two or three days.

Use the Food Guide Pyramid to plan meals, and check the "Look For" lists in Chapter 4 for menu ideas and an expanded range of healthful choices.

Be flexible and plan to take advantage of seasonal items. For example, although you may write down zucchini on your list, you may actually choose crookneck or another summer squash variety because the quality is exceptional and the price is right.

In the United States, especially in large supermarkets, we can purchase almost any fruit and vegetable at any time of the year. The highest quality and lowest price for each variety is available during and at the end of its peak growing season. At that time you are likely to see larger quantities of that fruit or vegetable on display and often there will be advertised sales.

To promote variety and to find new flavors you and your family might enjoy, choose several varieties of a fresh fruit or vegetable that is in season. For example, rather than buying four plums or apples, buy one each of four different plums or four different apples and do a home taste comparison.

When making your list, check your refrigerator, freezer, and cupboard to make sure you are not duplicating items you already have. Plan to buy a few impulse items each week—new things to try, snacks that aren't part of your plan, or items that are a better value than what you planned to buy. But try to limit your impulse purchases overall. Impulse items usually come at a premium price—in money, calories, fat, or all three. Try to shop after you have eaten a meal. Impulse purchases are more tempting to hungry shoppers.

Coupons and Rebates

Clip coupons and rebate certificates for products you buy regularly. You'll find them in magazines, newspaper supplements, mailbox flyers, supermarket shelf dispensers, and register tapes.

At the store, compare similar products and package sizes to determine which is the most economical choice. Less-advertised brands, store brands, generic products, or sale items can be less expensive than the branded item with a cents-off coupon. Sometimes, you may prefer a particular brand for its flavor, texture, or some other quality. But when a coupon for another brand offers a significant price advantage, why not give it a try? After trying both products, you can make a more informed choice the next time.

Organize all coupons by product type (salad dressing, frozen pizza, etc.) and put them in order with highest values and those expiring soonest at the beginning of each category. Store coupons often are good only for a few days; manufacturers' coupons usually allow a longer time to buy the product. You may want to use a coupon organizer, paper clips, or envelopes.

Manufacturers and supermarkets issue coupons to build sales and brand loyalty. Some stores promote double or even triple coupons; others limit coupon use to one or two purchases per coupon. Regardless of your store's policies, don't waste time clipping or saving coupons for products that you will never use.

If possible, multiply your savings by using a coupon and mail-in proof of purchase for a rebate for the same product. Refunds and rebates may be in the form of cash, check, a coupon to be used on a future purchase, or a free product sample. Usually, you must mail in a coupon, register receipt, and/or a universal product code seal (bar code) or other packaging to get a rebate. Remember that you are paying postage and supplying an envelope, so obtaining the rebate costs you about 40 cents and it will take several weeks or months to receive. Make sure the rebate is worth your time and effort.

Look for rebate offers not only in newspapers and magazines but also on supermarket bulletin boards, at customer service counters, and on end-of-aisle displays. Some coupon books and value packs will come in the mail. Toll-free customer service lines may add you to their rebate mailing list.

In-Store Sales

Most stores have some foods on sale at special prices. Depending on store size and advertising budget, special prices may be promoted in circulars or newspapers. Many stores offer samples of new or selected products and offer a sale price on the item. Take advantage of the opportunities to taste-test new items before you buy them. When you see an item at a favorable price, consider substituting it for a similar food on your shopping list. Stock up and buy several cans or packages of frozen or canned foods during special sales—but only if you use that food regularly.

Over half of shoppers use frequent shopper programs or savings clubs weekly. Frequent shopper programs offer special prices to patrons who present a customer recognition card. This system gives stores an opportunity to track purchases and gives shoppers additional discounts for shopping regularly at a preferred store or chain. Often, the total amount saved appears on the register tape.

Some stores have "buy one–get one free," two-for-one specials, such as two 5-pound bags of potatoes for the price of one. Shop with a friend and divide the bounty and price, especially if you won't use 10 pounds of potatoes within a week or two. If you get a second item free, and don't expect to use it soon, try to prolong its value to you. For example, sauté and freeze a second package of mushrooms for use later.

Some shoppers go to several stores, selecting the discounted items at each. Consider the value of your time and the cost of mileage. Is an extra 30 or 40 minutes of shopping and transportation time worth more or less than the potential in savings?

Watch for discount value days or for senior discounts if you are eligible for them. Some stores have special days that benefit a worthy organization with a certain percentage of sales. You can support schools, community groups, or charities by doing your shopping on those days.

Working the Aisles

You've probably heard it before, but it's worth repeating: Eat first, then shop. Don't shop when you are hungry or rushed—

those are the times you are more likely to indulge in expensive impulse purchases. If time is at a premium, shop when stores aren't crowded—early in the morning, late in the evening, or midweek rather than on weekends. Some stores are open around the clock; others have limited service hours.

Remember that store brands and generic food packages are usually less expensive than national brands, but they vary in quality. Some stores may have a regular brand and a premium one. Take a moment to check nutritional information, ingredients, and size of package. The only way to compare flavor and texture, though, is to try it. Some stores offer samples of new items or foods being promoted. This gives you a chance to taste before spending money on a new food or brand.

There are many foods that provide similar nutrients at widely varying cost levels. By making a decision to select the lowest-priced options, you can achieve substantial savings every time you shop.

To get the most for your food dollar, compare different forms of a food. For example, chicken breasts (typically $2.69 per pound) are far more costly than a whole chicken (typically 79 cents to $1.29 per pound). Expect to pay 10 to 20 cents more per pound for chicken that has been quartered or cut-up. A sharp knife or cleaver and about two minutes can save you more than 50 cents on a 3 1/2-pound chicken. Buy three or four whole chickens when the price is favorable and cut them up. Bag similar pieces in freezer bags in the amount you will cook in one meal or recipe.

Similarly, shredded cheese is more costly than solid cheese. Is the convenience worth the extra money? Can you easily slice or shred cheese at home to save $1.00 or more per pound? Pecan halves are usually more expensive than chopped or broken pecans. As a garnish, you may want halves; but broken or chopped nuts may be fine for cookies or in salads.

Also compare package sizes. Unit prices are usually higher for small packages. Some stores have shelf markers that tell you price per unit. The unit may be an ounce, a quart, or another measure. The best buy is the lowest price per unit. For example, a 22-ounce pizza at $4.79 (22 cents per ounce) is a better value than a popular brand of deluxe pizza in the 12-ounce size at $3.29 (27 cents per ounce). The store brand on sale for $2.50 for a 22-ounce pizza (11 cents per ounce) is the best choice in terms of price. For shelf stable foods, like rice or pasta, buying a larger size usually makes sense. But buy the economy or family packs only if you can use the whole amount before the food spoils or must be discarded. Buying economy packs of frequently used nonfood items like paper towels or cleaning supplies can save money and is a good strategy if you have space to store them.

Buy only the amount you will need—especially of fresh and perishable food. Purchasing deli foods by weight and purchasing cereal, dried fruit, or nuts from the bulk food section gives you control over amounts. Talk to the person at the meat counter or in the produce section if you want a smaller amount of prepackaged meat or produce. They should be willing to split and repackage a 4-pack of chops or split a bunch of parsley. Buy only as much dried spice and herbs as you will use in a few months; they lose flavor and pungency in prolonged storage. If you need just a little of a vegetable for a recipe, check out the salad bar. It costs more per pound, but you can buy 1/4 or 1/2 cup of sliced mushrooms or peppers for a stir-fry and have no waste.

At the checkout counter, pay attention to the price as the cashier scans each item. Be sure that you are getting the food at prices posted on in-store sales and on packages. Sometimes the price scanned is not the correct or current price. Remember to present coupons for items purchased before the checker begins checking your order. Buying groceries with some credit cards can earn frequent flyer miles. Earning frequent flyer miles makes sense only if you pay off your credit card balance each month, because interest charges will quickly erase any savings.

If your store doesn't carry something you want, ask for it. Many stores will make an effort to supply items or brands their patrons are seeking. The grocery business is very competitive. Consumers will be spending about half a trillion dollars in supermarkets by the year 2000. Remember, you're the customer, and pleasing customers is what keeps stores in business.

The Price of Convenience

Many people are willing to pay more for the convenience of pre-cut and prepared foods that save time and effort in the kitchen. Prepared foods to carry out or to heat and eat are one of the fastest growing supermarket categories. Although these "home meal replacement" products usually cost more, they save shopping and cooking time, have no waste, and minimize clean-up. If your goal is a quick, healthy meal with no mess, these "value-added" products offer great advantages. You'll find an ever-increasing array of value-added products in the fresh fruit and vegetable section of the store, such as bags of shredded carrots, fresh-squeezed juices, and cut, fresh pineapple. These alternatives are labor-free (for you) but command premium prices. For example, at one store, a pound of fresh carrots costs 59 cents; a bag of shredded carrots costs $1.89 for 8 ounces, or $3.78 per pound. Clearly if you have a few minutes to peel and shred plain carrots, you can save a lot of money.

Almost every store sells stalks of celery as well as bags of celery hearts. At one store, celery is 69 cents per pound, while celery hearts are $1.99. The economical choice is very clear. The large, outer stalks of celery can be used for chopping or for celery sticks.

Some premium-priced, value-added foods save only a few minutes of washing or preparation time. For example, a 3-ounce container of cinnamon sugar for making cinnamon toast costs 93 cents. Mixing ground cinnamon and sugar together takes less than a minute; you probably have both ingredients in your pantry. Three ounces of the homemade mix costs only about 9 cents.

Buying a few ounces or a single serving of mixed ingredients from a salad bar is more costly than buying, cleaning, and combining ingredients; however, there is no waste and your choice is packaged and ready-to-eat. But paying salad bar prices of $2.50 or $2.89 a pound for lettuce or spinach that is just washed and torn is generally a poor value. Bags of ready-to-eat mixed salad greens packaged with a gas that maintains their freshness can cost even more—$1.99 to $2.99 for an 8- to 10-ounce bag (about $4.44 per pound).

Buying frozen, loose-packed fruits and vegetables in plastic bags is often an economical choice. (It's harder to use only part of a boxed fruit or vegetable that is in a frozen "brick.") You can pour out only what you need, reseal the bag, and return it to the freezer. Individually quick-frozen berries, peaches, and melon balls usually keep their shape and texture better if eaten while slightly frozen.

Single-serving packages of juices, cereals, yogurt, puddings, snacks, etc., are almost always more costly than the same food purchased in a larger container. Foods for single people and small families tend to carry premium prices. But additional packaging costs may be justified by a product's convenience and portability for lunch boxes and briefcases. Most of the time, however, pouring juice or scooping pudding from a larger container is the economical choice—as long as you can use the entire package while the food is of good quality.

Carbonated beverages are far more economical in 2-liter bottles than in 12-ounce cans or bottles. Once opened, however, they must be used fairly soon. Unless several glasses will be poured, single serving cans are usually a better choice because the quality and flavor remain intact in unopened cans.

Shopping from Home

Some stores have services that allow patrons to call or fax in orders and have the groceries delivered. A new option in some communities is on-line grocery-shopping services in partnership with local markets. This shop-at-home service can save time and is convenient especially if you have a computer and aren't one who feels the need to see, touch, and smell food before you buy it. For people who are homebound and for others who prefer their groceries to be delivered, on-line shopping is a plus. You should expect to pay additional fees for on-line time, delivery, and other electronic services, though. The service lists foods with prices so comparisons can be made and economical choices selected. Some programs will show you nutrition labels and ingredient lists to allow product comparisons. Some on-line services also offer weekly specials and coupons.

Recycling and Environmental Issues

The American Dietetic Association advocates personal and community-based activities to protect the environment and conserve natural resources. Many food and other products sold in the supermarket come in cans, bottles, bags, and other packages that can be recycled.

Do your part by recycling. Some plastic and foil containers and glass jars can be reused several times in your home kitchen or as storage containers. Choose products sold in containers that can be recycled and take advantage of recycling programs at your supermarket and in your community.

Chapter Four

Up and Down
the Aisles

WHETHER IT'S A NEIGHBORHOOD GROCERY STORE or mega supermarket, there are plenty of choices when you shop for food.

Here, in bite-sized pieces, we present information that will help you be an informed shopper. Organized in food groups based on the Food Guide Pyramid, you'll discover the key products or attributes to "Look For" as you make your way down the aisles. Then, we provide more general tips that "Shoppers Should Know"—advice that will help you become a savvy shopper. Through it all, you'll get the information you need to make the healthiest choices for you and your family.

Breads and Bread Products

Look For

- ➤ Whole-grain or multigrain breads and rolls with whole wheat, cracked wheat, spelt, oat, millet, or other whole grains as the first ingredient on the ingredient list.
- ➤ Enriched white breads and rolls.
- ➤ Breads, rolls, and muffins with 3 grams of fat or less per serving, including soft or crisp bread sticks, bagels, bialys, English muffins, lavosh, flatbreads, matzo, crumpets, pita bread, and soft corn or flour tortillas.
- ➤ Breads and muffins made with wheat bran, oat bran, or added pea fiber; bread products labeled "high in fiber" or "good source of fiber."

Source: U.S. Department of Agriculture/U.S. Department of Health and Human Services, 1992.

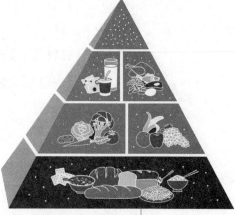

Bread, Cereal, Rice, & Pasta in The Food Guide Pyramid

Bread, Cereal, Rice, & Pasta
6-11 servings

• Fat (naturally occurring and added)   △ Sugars (added)

➤ Pita pockets, especially whole-grain ones. Fill them for sandwiches or toast them to make snack crackers for dips.
➤ Ready-made pizza crusts, including whole-wheat ones, for homemade pizza.
➤ Frozen or chilled pizza crust; Italian and French bread dough.
➤ Canned New England brown bread with molasses, whole-wheat, and raisins.
➤ Frozen low-fat waffles and pancakes, including whole-grain varieties.

Shoppers Should Know

The date on the label is a clue to freshness. Packaged bakery products usually have a longer shelf life than homemade items or ones baked in the in-store bakery.

Whole-wheat flour is made from the whole grain including the wheat germ and wheat bran. It is fuller-flavored, has more fiber and is more nutritious than all-purpose flour.

Wheat breads that don't specify whole wheat on the ingredient label are usually made from refined white flour. The first ingredient listed on the label is the primary grain. Some breads have added caramel (brown) color.

Rye and pumpernickel breads, although brown, contain primarily white flour. They are not whole-grain breads.

Enriched breads have the thiamin, niacin, riboflavin, and iron lost during the flour-refining process restored to them. They are more nutritious than unenriched white breads but lack most of the fiber, chromium, copper, magnesium, zinc, vitamin B6, and vitamin E of whole-grain breads. Folate added to enriched flour makes white breads a good source of folate.

Calcium propionate is an additive (with an excellent safety record) often used to keep bread products fresh longer. The additive provides some additional calcium.

Breads made with recipes that contain no fat (like traditional French or Italian bread) and those without preservatives become stale faster. Buy small loaves that can be used within a day or two. Store them at room temperature in a tightly closed bag. Cut stale bread into cubes and toast for croutons or to make bread crumbs.

Some breads labeled as light use refined cellulose (wood pulp) to provide added fiber. Because refined cellulose is not digested, it provides no calories. Refined cellulose does not carry with it several of the nutrients that accompany the fiber in whole grains.

Prepared garlic bread is usually quite high in fat and carries a premium price. Scrape off excess fat before heating it or make your own by brushing margarine or oil and garlic on French or Italian bread.

Challah and egg breads contain egg yolks and are sources of dietary cholesterol.

Bakery breads often don't have nutrition labeling. Look at the ingredient list to see what fats, flours, and sugars are used.

Some bread products are fortified with calcium. Check the label.

Most biscuits, croissants, scones, doughnuts, sweet rolls, cheese breads, and focaccias are high in fat.

"Giant" muffins, rolls, and biscuits can have four times the calories and fat as regular-sized ones. Look for small muffins, rolls, and biscuits or make your own with reduced-fat mixes or from recipes with little fat.

Flaky bread sticks that are layered twists of dough made with butter contain lots of fat to make and keep them flaky.

Frozen phyllo dough is fat-free. Most recipes call for brushing butter or margarine between layers. You can substitute butter-flavored spray.

Canned, chilled biscuit and roll doughs generally have 5 to 8 grams fat per biscuit or roll.

Lime-treated corn uses calcium chloride to help remove the tough outer hull of corn. This treatment, often used in making traditional corn tortillas, provides extra calcium and improves the protein quality. Most soft corn tortillas sold in supermarkets have little calcium. Check the Nutrition Facts panel.

Traditional fried corn tortilla, tostado, and taco shells are fried in lard. Soft flour and corn tortillas usually have little or no fat. Read ingredient panels to check the type of fat used and the Nutrition Facts panel to see the amount of fat. Choose baked, fat-free, or soft tortillas and similar products most of the time.

Folate, a B vitamin, helps cells divide normally and helps protect against birth defects. There is some medical evidence that increasing folate protects against heart disease. Folate added to enriched flour makes white bread and pasta good sources of folate.

Packaged plain bread crumbs have added salt, 185 to 225 milligrams per 1/4 cup. If sodium is a concern, make soft bread crumbs from leftover bread using a food processor or blender for immediate use. If you plan to keep bread crumbs on the shelf, toast the bread before crushing it for crumbs.

Wheat-free breads for individuals sensitive to the gluten in wheat include corn tortillas, rice bread, and breads and rolls made with 100 percent rye or spelt flour. Carefully read labels because many breads contain several grains even though the main label may say rye or millet bread.

Baking Mixes

Look For

➤ Angel food cake mix.

➤ Light or reduced-fat mixes for cakes, brownies, cookies, and desserts.

➤ Whole-grain bread and muffin mixes.

➤ Low-fat quickbread and biscuit mixes.

➤ Pancake and waffle mixes that can be prepared without added fat, including buttermilk, buckwheat, Swedish, and blueberry varieties, or buy low-fat frozen waffles and pancakes.

➤ Pizza crust mixes and prepared pizza crusts that have 3 grams of fat or less per serving.

Shoppers Should Know

Most mixes have a two-column Nutrition Facts panel listing both mix alone and baked (prepared) values. The "as prepared" nutrient values are the important ones because they include the ingredients (usually fat, eggs, or milk) used in preparation.

Packaged stuffing mixes are usually low in fat, but the instructions say to add lots of margarine. Add half the recommended amount of margarine and some extra liquid or chopped vegetables for flavor and moistness. To boost calcium intake, replace half of the broth or water in stuffing mix recipes with skim or low-fat milk.

Two egg whites or 1/4 cup of egg substitute can be used to replace each egg called for in baking mixes. Mashed banana, applesauce, prune purée, or tofu can replace eggs in some products such as muffins. When replacing eggs or fat in a recipe, choose an ingredient that has a flavor compatible with the recipe and expect some difference in texture.

Packaged bread mixes for breadmakers command premium prices, often as much as bakery breads.

Cereal

Look For

- ➤ Whole-grain cooked and ready-to-eat cereals such as oatmeal and shredded wheat. They're economical and nutrient-rich.
- ➤ Cereals with at least 3 grams of fiber and 3 grams or less of fat per serving.
- ➤ Vitamin-and-mineral-fortified cereals. Most supply 25% Daily Value for key vitamins and minerals. Some provide 100% Daily Value making them comparable to a multivitamin and mineral supplement pill.
- ➤ Cereals with a grain as the first ingredient on the ingredient list.
- ➤ Low-fat, grain-based cereal and fruit bars. They make a portable, nutritious breakfast or snack.
- ➤ Grain-fruit-nut cereals with whole grains and dried fruits listed as the first three ingredients on the ingredient list.
- ➤ Toasted wheat germ, wheat bran, or oat bran to add fiber and nutrients to recipes.

Shoppers Should Know

The date on the box is a guide to shelf life.

Cereals aren't just for breakfast. They can be enjoyed as a light meal or snack, too.

Cereals that have sugar, honey, corn syrup, fructose, molasses, fruit juice sweetener, or malt syrup as the first ingredient contain more sugar than grain.

Eight grams of sugar per serving in a presweetened cereal is equivalent to one rounded spoonful of sugar, the amount many people add from the sugar bowl. If you would sweeten your cereal anyway, there is no reason to avoid presweetened varieties.

Wheat bran is only one of many beneficial fibers. Oats, oat bran, corn bran, and fruit and bean fibers offer heart-healthy benefits; wheat bran promotes regularity.

Wheat germ is rich in folate and other vitamins and minerals. Adding wheat germ to recipes adds a bit of crunch and boosts nutrients. Try it in meat loaves and casseroles, and mixed with bread crumbs whenever bread crumbs are used.

Granola-type cereals, muesli, and cereals with nuts or coconut usually have more fat than plain grain cereals. Reduced- and low-fat granola-type cereals are available.

Fortified cereals usually cost more than nonfortified ones. Because many of the vitamins and minerals in fortified cereals are sprayed on, be sure to drink all the milk left in the bottom of the bowl.

Oatmeal comes in many forms, each with different cooking times and different textures. Some refined types just require the addition of boiling water or 2 minutes of cooking. Steel-cut oats cook in 30 minutes.

Flavored hot cereals may contain added fat and sugar. Instant hot cereals are higher in sodium than regular cooked varieties. Read the labels.

Grits, cream of wheat, and cream of rice are refined grains and have little fiber.

Some cereals, including some brans and granolas, contain saturated fat or partially hydrogenated fat that can raise your blood cholesterol levels. Check the ingredient list and Nutrition Facts panel.

If artificial colors, flavors, sweeteners, or preservatives in cereal are of concern to you, look on the ingredient list to see if these additives are present. BHA, BHT, and TBHQ are added to some cereals as antioxidants and preservatives to maintain their freshness and crispness.

Pasta, Rice, and Grains

Look For

- ➤ All pasta, rice, and grain products.
- ➤ Pasta in all forms, including whole-wheat pasta.
- ➤ Grains including couscous, cornmeal, bulgur, buckwheat, barley, oatmeal, oat bran, quinoa, grits, kasha, cracked wheat, wheat germ, amaranth, kamut, millet, spelt, teff, triticale, wild rice, and brown rice for added nutrients and fiber.
- ➤ Lasagna, ravioli, tortellini, and manicotti filled with part-skim ricotta cheese.

Shoppers Should Know

Omitting salt from cooking water for pasta and rice reduces sodium intake.

Fresh pastas cook more quickly than dried pastas but are usually more expensive and should be used within two days of purchase.

Most dried pasta is egg free, with the exception of noodles. Egg noodles have 55 to 70 milligrams of cholesterol per serving. If cholesterol is a problem, choose yolk-free noodles. Fresh pasta is usually made with eggs.

To cut fat, serve pasta with tomato- and vegetable-based sauces instead of butter- and cream-based sauces. Try salsa to season pasta, rice, and grains.

Filled pasta entrées may contain cheese or meat fillings or sauces that are high in fat.

Frozen pasta entrées are often high in fat and sodium. Read labels and compare.

When pastas cook, they usually double in volume. When rice cooks, it usually triples in volume.

Pasta salad from salad bars and pasta salad mixes often contain high-fat dressing. Check out those with light dressings.

Packaged macaroni and cheese mixes carry dual nutrition labeling—as packaged and as prepared. Look at the prepared values and the size of portion stated. Packaged macaroni and cheese is more economical than macaroni and cheese prepared from scratch. Most macaroni and cheese is high in sodium, whether from a mix, frozen, or prepared from scratch. Fat levels vary depending upon the cheese and other ingredients used.

Brown rice has almost three times the fiber of white rice.

Quick-cooking grains and seasoned grain mixes save time but are higher in sodium and usually carry premium prices.

Many grain and pasta mixes call for added margarine. Use only half the seasoning packet and half the amount of margarine. To save money and reduce fat, add herbs, vegetables, or low-sodium broths to season plain rice or pasta.

Gluten-free grains include amaranth, buckwheat, cornmeal, millet, quinoa, rice, teff, and wild rice.

Oriental bifun noodles are made with white rice flour and

potato starch; saifun noodles with mung bean starch; soba noodles with buckwheat starch.

Ramen noodles are sold in individual blocks with seasoning packets in many flavors, most with flavor-enhancing additives. To reduce sodium, use only half of the flavor packet. Check the Nutrition Facts panel for amounts of sodium and fat.

Crackers

Look For

➤ Crackers that are fat-free and low-fat (3 grams of fat or less per serving), such as rice, oat, or barley cakes; melba toast; saltines; lavosh; whole-grain flatbreads; matzo; wheat thins; pepper crackers; whole-grain wafers and imported wafer crackers; flavored crispbreads; and oyster crackers.

➤ Whole-grain crispbreads. They are low-fat or fat-free, cholesterol-free, and provide valuable fiber.

➤ Crackers you regularly choose in a reduced-fat or low-sodium version.

➤ Seeded crackers for a little extra fiber.

Shoppers Should Know

To check the Nutrition Facts panel for the number of crackers per serving and the calorie, fat, fiber, and sugars content.

The words "flaky," "rich" or "croissant" on the label usually mean the crackers are made with extra fat. Cheese crackers also tend to have additional fat.

Fat-free does not mean healthy or low-calorie. Calorie levels of some fat-free crackers are not much lower than regular varieties. Compare labels.

Smaller servings of regular cracker varieties are fine if you prefer the taste over the low-fat, fat-free, or low-sodium varieties.

Many crackers are made with butter, coconut and palm oils, vegetable shortening, or hydrogenated oils. Check the ingredient list and the amount of saturated fat listed on the Nutrition Facts panel.

Cookies, Bars, and Snack Cakes

Look For

> ➤ Low-fat cookies with moderate amounts of sugar, such as graham crackers, animal crackers, arrowroot cookies, zwieback, gingersnaps, vanilla wafers, biscotti, and fruit-filled bars (such as fig bars).
> ➤ Small or single-serving cupcakes, doughnuts, and sweet rolls, instead of jumbo sizes.
> ➤ Granola bars, particularly low-fat ones and those without lots of peanut butter or chocolate, for a portable snack, dessert, or breakfast.
> ➤ Cookies, brownies, and bars that are reduced-fat, low-fat, or fat-free.
> ➤ Meringue cookies, baked meringue, dessert shells, and lady fingers. They are fat-free.

Shoppers Should Know

The Nutrition Facts panel on the label states the number of cookies per serving. All calorie and nutrient levels are based on that number of cookies.

When comparing cookies, it's important for you to check the label to see how many cookies are listed as a serving. About 1 ounce of cookies is a standard serving. Some manufacturers, however, label 1 cookie (0.6 oz.) as a serving, making it look like a lower calorie choice. Be sure to double the calorie value if you eat two of these very small cookies.

Fat-free does not mean healthy or low-calorie. Calorie levels may be similar to regular varieties because additional sugar may be added.

Smaller servings of regular cookie varieties are fine if you prefer the taste over that of low-fat or fat-free varieties.

Many cookies are made with butter, coconut and palm oils, vegetable shortening, or partially hydrogenated oils. Check the ingredient list and amount of saturated fat listed on the Nutrition Facts panel.

Read the labels on frozen and refrigerated cookie doughs. Some brands have only 2 1/2 grams of fat per cookie while others have 12 grams of fat per cookie.

Toaster pastries are generally made from refined flour, fat, sugar, preserves, and artificial colors and flavors. This means they are not good sources of essential nutrients and fiber. There are reduced-fat pastries available.

Energy bars are used by athletes but many non-athletes eat them as snacks. Most energy bars contain at least 60 percent of calories from carbohydrates; most have 200 to 300 calories; many are vitamin- and mineral-fortified. If you are limiting your calorie and fat intake, choose a bar that contains less than 225 calories and less than 3 grams of fat per bar.

Packaged Snack Foods

Most packaged snacks are grain-based but some are from the fruit or vegetable food groups. Most are discussed here.

Look For

➤ Already-popped popcorn or unpopped popcorn without added fat for air poppers or microwave ovens. They have 3 grams of fat or less per 3-cup serving.

➤ Rice and popcorn cakes, which are available in many flavors.

➤ Fat-free, reduced-fat, or low-fat corn, tortilla, vegetable, or potato chips or crisps. Some are baked, some made with less fat, and still others made with a type of fat that cannot be absorbed.

➤ Whole-grain, low-fat snack chips.

➤ Unsalted pretzels, which are also low in fat. Even salted pretzels are lower in fat and sodium than most other salty snacks.

➤ Fat-free or low-fat caramel corn, corn puffs, or cheese puffs.

➤ Small boxes or bags of raisins, trail mix, cereal mixes, and other fruit and nut combinations.

Shoppers Should Know

Many snack items are high in calories, fat, sodium, and/or sugar and have minimal nutritional value. Substitute fresh fruit or raw vegetables for fried or sweet snacks some of the time.

Fat-free potato chips made with olestra, a non-absorbable fat, have half the calories of regular chips and taste like traditional potato chips. Some people report mild gastrointestinal symptoms after eating these snacks, especially in excess. If these, or any other foods, cause distress, either omit them from your diet or limit amounts eaten.

Individual (1-ounce) snack packs help to control portion size. Transferring snacks from larger packages to small plastic sandwich bags to make single servings reduces cost per serving— but may increase temptation to eat several "portions."

Candy, pastries, and chips in small, single-serving packages are good occasional treats. Eat them after you've met recommended servings from the various food groups.

Most brands of bagel and pita chips contain partially hydrogenated oils to retain crispness. A small (1-ounce) serving contains about 4 grams of fat. A fairly small (6-ounce) bag of bagel chips provides six servings.

One brand of apple chips has 4 grams of fat per ounce. Banana chips are both fried and sweetened. Check the Nutrition Facts panel for the fat and calorie content of all fruit chips.

Doughnuts vary in size and all are fried. If you eat doughnuts, choose small doughnuts to keep fat in check.

Fat-free or low-fat dips, salad dressings, and salsas keep veggies and fat-free and low-fat chips low in fat.

Source: U.S. Department of Agriculture/U.S. Department of Health and Human Services, 1992.

Vegetables
in The Food Guide Pyramid

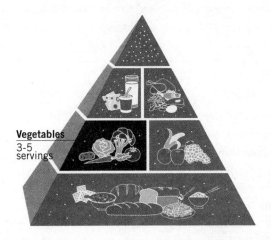

Vegetables
3-5
servings

• Fat (naturally occurring and added)   △ Sugars (added)

Fresh Vegetables

Look For

➤ Dark green, deep yellow, or orange-colored fresh vegetables (such as spinach or winter squash) and plan to eat at least one each day.

➤ Fresh vegetables that are in season. Many vegetables are available year-round, but quality and flavor are at their peak when vegetables are locally grown and abundant.

➤ Tomatoes in various sizes, shapes, and colors. Tomatoes should be firm, plump, smooth, and brightly colored with a clear skin. When ripe, tomatoes are firm but yield to gentle pressure.

➤ Small or medium-size colorful carrots that are crisp and smooth with pointy, firm tips. Fresh carrots have greens attached but carrot greens are inedible and must be discarded. Very large carrots are less sweet but good in soups or stock. Peeled and cut, baby and shredded carrots are convenient but carry premium prices.

Up and Down the Aisles

➤ Any type of cabbage: red, green, Chinese, Napa, etc. All should be heavy and solid with unbruised, firm heads.

➤ Green, red, yellow, and other bell (sweet) peppers. They should be plump, glossy, and unblemished. All are very rich in vitamin C; red and yellow peppers have more beta-carotene than green peppers.

➤ Crisp stalks of broccoli and broccoli rabe that are firm and bright green with compact clusters of dark green buds and no yellow or dry patches.

➤ Mushrooms that are fairly clean with tightly closed caps and no dried-out, spongy, or pitted surfaces. Use mushrooms within two days.

➤ Ever-popular potatoes in all forms, which provide complex carbohydrate, vitamin C, and some minerals. Potatoes should be firm, unbruised, dry, and free of cuts. Avoid potatoes with a greenish cast, grey spots, or sprouts.

➤ Freshly picked ears of corn—they're the sweetest. Choose ones with plump, cool-to-touch kernels. Avoid corn with hard or shriveled kernels.

➤ Fresh herbs to flavor your food. Buy pots of herbs for your garden or windowsill.

➤ A variety of salad greens, including deep green leafy ones for salads and sandwiches. Lettuce should be crisp in texture with no brown or soft spots and unblemished edges on the leaves. Iceberg lettuce should have a solid, crisp, tightly-packed head.

➤ Onions, garlic, and ginger—terrific flavor boosters with some health benefits. Onions, shallots, and garlic should be firm, dry, and well-shaped, free of sprouts or dark spots. Store them in a cool dry place but do not refrigerate. Gingerroot should be a fresh-looking firm root. A small root has a more delicate flavor than a large root. Break off a section that is the amount you wish to buy.

➤ Bags of sprouts such as bean sprouts, broccoli sprouts, radish sprouts, and alfalfa sprouts to add crunch and nutrients to salads and sandwiches.

➤ Crisp celery in unscarred bunches with fresh-looking

green leaves. Small stalks and celery hearts are more tender but much more expensive.

➤ Cucumbers that are firm, clear-skinned, and dark green. Choose slender ones, fairly thin in diameter, so there is more flesh and fewer seeds.

➤ Vegetables that are good sources of beta-carotene/vitamin A: dandelion; mustard, turnip, and collard greens; spinach; broccoli; beets; bok choy; carrots; kale; red bell peppers; winter squash; sweet potatoes; Swiss chard; tomatoes; calabasa pumpkin; and sugar snap peas.

➤ Vegetables that are good sources of vitamin C: green, red, and yellow bell peppers; tomatoes; Brussels sprouts; asparagus; broccoli; cabbage; cauliflower; spinach; kale; turnips; potatoes; mustard and collard greens; kohlrabi; snow peas; sugar snap peas; lotus root; potatoes; rutabagas; and sweet potatoes.

➤ Vegetables that are good sources of folate: asparagus, broccoli, okra, beets, artichokes, green peas, sugar snap peas, leeks, cauliflower, okra, parsnips, corn, lima beans, and all green leafy vegetables, such as spinach, cabbage, Brussels sprouts, romaine, leaf lettuce, chicory, escarole, beet greens, and turnip greens.

➤ Vegetables that are especially high in fiber: corn; artichokes; lima beans, baked beans, and other legumes; peas; winter squash; Brussels sprouts; and plantains.

➤ Vegetables that may help reduce the risk of cancer: cruciferous vegetables including collard, mustard, and turnip greens; Brussels sprouts; bok choy; broccoli, broccoli sprouts, and broccoli rabe; kohlrabi; cabbage; cauliflower; kale; and rutabaga.

➤ Vegetables that are good sources of vitamin E and calcium: deep green leafy vegetables such as spinach, kale, mustard greens, and turnip greens.

Shoppers Should Know

Although raw vegetables may not have nutrition labels, all are healthy choices. They are exempt from the requirement that all foods called healthy have a minimum of 10 percent of a key nutrient.

Beta-carotene is a substance that converts to an active form of vitamin A in the body. It is characteristically a yellow color and is present in yellow and orange vegetables and fruits, particularly carrots, winter squash, and sweet potatoes.

Buying fresh vegetables allows you to control the amount of added salt and fat used in preparation.

Store whole tomatoes at room temperature to maximize flavor; refrigerate cut tomatoes. Vine-ripened tomatoes are the most flavorful. Genetically engineered tomatoes have an extended shelf life when ripe.

Cabbage has many health benefits and is usually one of the least expensive vegetables.

Lettuces that are deep green have more vitamins than light green lettuces.

Eat corn as soon as possible after picking as it loses sweetness during storage.

Herb plants provide an ongoing supply at less cost than cut herbs by the ounce or bag. Fresh herbs are more flavorful, colorful, and aromatic than dried ones. Use herbs to add flavor to your cooking without adding fat or salt. Parsley, cilantro, and dill are the most economical herbs year-round. In the summer, enjoy bountiful basil, mint, rosemary, chives, and other varieties.

Washed, cut raw vegetables are a handy, low-calorie snack. Keep a jar or plastic bag of them in sight in your refrigerator. Reach for them often.

Most light-colored vegetables (iceberg lettuce, jicama, fennel, radishes, zucchini, celery, and cucumbers) have few nutrients but are good low-calorie fillers and munchies.

Precut vacuum-sealed salad greens are ready-to-use and convenient but command premium prices.

Organically grown fruits and vegetables meet varying criteria based on state regulations. Certification standards are based on the length of time the soil has been kept free from pesticides, herbicides, and contaminants from nonorganic fields. Organic foods are processed, transported, and stored without artificial preservatives, colorings, or irradiation. Earth-friendly food production may yield better tasting produce, but appearance and size of fruits and vegetables is less consistent, and the price of organic produce is often higher. Some supermarkets offer a wide variety of organic produce. Others offer a small selection at premium prices.

To enjoy their flavors and textures, vegetables should be prepared simply. Use minimal amounts of fats to enhance them.

Cut vegetables from the salad bar, ready-to-use spinach and mixed greens, and shredded carrots and cabbage reduce meal preparation time.

Some vegetables (broccoli, cabbage, kale, turnip greens, and collards) contain iron, but it is not absorbed as well as the iron in meats.

Buy only the amount of vegetables that you can use. When possible, split packs or bunches, especially when produce is priced by the pound rather than by the bunch.

Blended torn salad greens from the salad bar are convenient but usually more expensive than heads or bunches of salad greens.

Baking potatoes and sweet potatoes already cleaned and wrapped to prepare in the microwave are handy but command a premium price.

Pick up information about fresh vegetables on signs, brochures, and recipe cards in the produce section.

When a vegetable is not in season, a frozen or canned form is usually more economical and better quality.

Leftover cooked, chilled beets, carrots, beans, asparagus, and other vegetables make great salads and healthy snacks. Prepare extra vegetables at mealtimes for salads and snacks the next day.

"Breathable" storage bags, plastic bags with tiny holes, help to slow spoilage of fresh produce.

Eating potatoes and eggplant with skins left on boosts fiber intake. Zucchini and okra also add a fiber bonus.

Some vegetables and fruits, such as cucumbers and some apples, are coated with an edible wax to help prevent moisture loss and reduce shriveling. Peel skin from waxed produce.

Broccoli, cauliflower, cabbage, Brussels sprouts, and other cruciferous vegetables, whether fresh or frozen, contain substances that help protect cells of the lungs and breasts from potential carcinogens. Diets high in antioxidants including beta-carotene, vitamin C, vitamin E, and some phytochemicals (see next paragraph), protect cells from substances formed by inflammation and other disease processes.

The specific protective effects of many substances found in fruits and vegetables are a subject of current research. Phytochemicals are components in foods that are not nutrients, but may provide health benefits. It appears that phytochemicals, present in many vegetables, prevent cell damage and neutralize potential cancer-causing agents. Identified phytochemicals include indoles, in cruciferous vegetables, that may reduce the risk of breast cancer, and allylic sulfides, in garlic, onions, leeks, and chives, that seem to stimulate cell enzymes that detoxify cancer-causing agents. Others include lycopene, present in red vegetables such as tomatoes and red peppers, which is a potent antioxidant with anti-cancer properties; terpenes, found in eggplant, also seem to produce enzymes that deactivate cancer-causing agents.

Science is identifying more and more protective phytochemicals in food. Because so many of them are found in vegetables, fruits, and grains, eating a wide variety of foods from these groups offers multiple, albeit not yet well-understood, health benefits.

Frozen Vegetables

Look For

> ➤ Plain frozen vegetables that are packed without sauces or breading.
> ➤ Frozen vegetables that are good sources of beta-carotene/ vitamin A: dandelion, mustard, turnip, and collard greens; spinach; broccoli; carrots; kale; red bell peppers; winter squash; sweet potatoes; and Swiss chard.
> ➤ Frozen vegetables that are good sources of vitamin C: green, red, and yellow bell peppers; Brussels sprouts; asparagus; broccoli; cauliflower; spinach; kale; beet, mustard and collard greens; snow peas; sugar snap peas; potatoes; and sweet potatoes.
> ➤ Frozen vegetables that are good sources of folate: asparagus, broccoli, okra, beets, artichokes, green peas, cauliflower, sugar snap peas, asparagus, Brussels sprouts, mixed

vegetable blends, and all green leafy vegetables, such as spinach.

➤ Vegetables that are especially high in fiber: corn, artichokes, lima beans, okra, peas, winter squash, and Brussels sprouts.

➤ Frozen vegetables rich in antioxidant vitamin E: deep green leafy vegetables such as spinach, kale, and turnip greens.

➤ Frozen cruciferous vegetables including collard, mustard and turnip greens, Brussels sprouts, broccoli, cauliflower, and kale, which may help reduce the risk of cancer.

Shoppers Should Know

Frozen vegetables are packed at their peak of freshness, so they are equal to fresh vegetables in nutrient content.

Plain (unseasoned) frozen vegetables allow you to control the amount of salt and fat added in preparation.

Most frozen vegetables with sauces are high in sodium and/or fat. Look at the Nutrition Facts panel of vegetables with cream or butter sauces.

Bags of frozen chopped onions, green and red peppers, and chives kept in the freezer are handy when you need small amounts for recipes.

Some vegetables contain iron, but it is not absorbed as well as iron in meats.

Frozen vegetables in 1-pound bags are usually an economical choice and save preparation time. Remove as much of the vegetable as you will use; seal the bag with a twist tie and return it to the freezer.

Frozen baked potatoes, zucchini, okra, and eggplant with edible seeds and/or skins add a fiber bonus.

Breaded onion rings, hash browns, French fries, cheese-topped potatoes, twice-baked potatoes, batter-coated zucchini, spinach and corn soufflés, green beans with mushroom sauce, creamed spinach, and vegetables with cheese sauce are likely to be higher in fat than other veggies. If you choose these, eat moderate portions.

Canned and Bottled Vegetables

Look For

➤ Canned and bottled vegetables. They are quick and convenient sources of many vitamins and minerals as well as fiber.

➤ Canned tomatoes: peeled whole, puréed, crushed, sauced, stewed, diced and seasoned with herbs or vegetables. All are nutrient-rich and usually less expensive than fresh tomatoes for most cooking uses.

➤ Bottles of tomato-based sauces with a variety of flavors and textures. They are great to keep on the pantry shelf for a quick meal over pasta, polenta, or cooked vegetables.

➤ Canned legumes (peas, beans, and lentils), which are time-savers, economical, and excellent sources of fiber, folate, protein, and iron (see page 78).

➤ Ethnic prepared foods in cans or jars, such as eggplant capanota, olive blends, Giardiniera, roasted red peppers, and stuffed grape leaves.

➤ Jars of chopped, minced, or roasted garlic. They are real time-savers. They must be refrigerated after opening.

➤ Tomato, vegetable, and carrot juices. Choose low-sodium versions if sodium is restricted. Vegetable juices may be purchased freshly extracted, frozen, or bottled.

➤ Bottled beet borscht, unless sodium is restricted.

➤ Salsa as a dip, for seasoning other foods, or to top baked potatoes.

➤ Prepared salads in jars—corn relish, three-bean salad, pickled beets, and marinated artichokes.

➤ Good sources of beta-carotene, a form of vitamin A: canned greens, spinach, beets, carrots, asparagus, roasted red peppers, sweet potatoes, and tomatoes.

➤ Good sources of folate: creamed corn, canned greens, spinach, artichoke hearts, asparagus, lima beans, baked beans, refried beans, kidney beans, great Northern beans, and peas.

Shoppers Should Know

All canned vegetables carry a Nutrition Facts panel.

Canned vegetables are similar in nutrient value to raw, frozen, and freshly cooked vegetables.

Canned single and mixed vegetables and fruits are all "healthy" according to the Food and Drug Administration's rules, whether or not they say it on the label.

Canned vegetables are precooked to retain texture and nutrients. To avoid overcooking, reheat with liquids from can just a few minutes until hot. Drained liquids from canned vegetables contain some nutrients and may be added to soup stock or sauces.

Many varieties of beans—baked beans, garbanzos (chickpeas), kidney, great Northern, red beans, butter beans, lima beans, and low-fat refried beans—come in cans. Drain and rinse beans before adding them to recipes if sodium is restricted. The liquid in the can contains salt to help keep beans firm.

Some canned vegetables can be combined to make easy salads or vegetarian entrées. Mix drained black beans with corn, and roasted red peppers with drained marinated artichokes.

Canned legumes such as baked beans, chickpeas, black-eyed peas, kidney beans, and black beans can be counted as servings from either the vegetable or the meat group in the Food Guide Pyramid.

If you need to restrict sodium, choose no-salt-added, low-sodium, or reduced-sodium canned vegetables.

Harvard or pickled beets and sweet and sour cabbage are generally low-fat or fat-free. Beets, especially pickled beets, are high in sodium.

Tomato juice, with just 40 calories per cup, is rich in vitamin C. Several recent studies have shown that tomato-rich diets are linked with lower incidence of stomach, prostate, and breast cancers, although confirmation is needed. Tomatoes contain a variety of protective nutrients and phytochemicals. And canned tomatoes, because of processing methods, are a more concentrated source of nutrients than fresh tomatoes.

Carrot juice contains many vitamins, phytochemicals, and fiber. Try cooking couscous or other grains in carrot juice for an interesting flavor and added nutrient content.

Sauerkraut, marinated artichokes, sweet and sour cabbage, pickled vegetables, and some seasoned tomatoes have more salt than other canned vegetables.

If a can of vegetables is swollen or bulging or shows evidence of discolored metal inside, the can should be discarded.

Even canned foods don't last forever. There are some flavor changes and quality losses over time. From time to time, check your pantry shelves and use cans of food that have been there for several months. Tomatoes and high-acid vegetables and fruits should be used within 18 months for optimum quality. Other vegetables should be used within two years.

Fresh Fruit
(including fresh juices/refrigerated fruits)

Look For

➤ Ripe, sweet fruit for use within a day or two; firm, less-ripe fruit to ripen at home for eating later in the week;

**Fruits
in The Food Guide Pyramid**

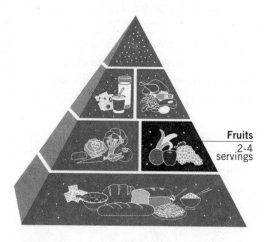

Fruits
2-4
servings

• Fat (naturally occurring and added)   Δ Sugars (added)

Source: U.S. Department of Agriculture/U.S. Department of Health and Human Services, 1992.

bargain-priced, bruised, or overripe fruit to chop and use in baking or to make fruit preserves or chutneys.

➤ Nutrition information about fresh fruits on signs and flyers in the produce section of your grocery store.

➤ Locally grown fruit in season. It's likely to be at peak flavor and a good buy.

➤ New varieties of fruits you may not have tried before, such as fresh mangos and papayas. Expand the range of healthful fruit you enjoy.

➤ Oranges, grapefruit, lemons, limes, and other citrus that have thin unblemished but firm skins and feel heavy in relation to size. Use citrus zest and juice to season grains, vegetables, and meat.

➤ Bananas that have clear unbruised skin that is (ripe) yellow or (unripe) light green. They will continue to ripen at home at room temperature. Never refrigerate bananas. Overripe bananas with black spots or dark skins are very sweet and can be used for baking.

➤ Red, green, and golden apples that are firm, bright-skinned and unbruised. Try different varieties of apples—many of the most tasty ones are not big, red, and shiny.

➤ Melons that are firm and unbruised. They continue to ripen at room temperature and then should be refrigerated. Cantaloupes and other small melons are ripe when they yield to gentle pressure at the stem end. Ask someone in the produce section to help you select a ripe melon until you can judge for yourself.

➤ Grapes that are firm, plump, and dry. They should adhere to stems and not be shriveled near the stem ends.

➤ Peaches that are firm, colorful, and unbruised. The shape, flavor, and size depend on the variety. Ripen at room temperature, then refrigerate. Ripe fruit yields to gentle pressure.

➤ Strawberries that are firm, dry, and uniformly dark red with fresh green caps. Size does not influence flavor. Avoid packages with any soggy berries or evidence of mold.

➤ Pineapples that are firm with a trace of orange color near the bottom. Pineapples do not ripen after picking.

Hawaiian pineapples are generally the sweetest. Store at room temperature, since pineapple blackens if refrigerated. If cut, refrigerate and use within two days.

➤ Good sources of vitamin C: kiwi, mangos, cantaloupe, cherimoya, papayas, guavas, honeydew melons, tangerines, oranges, grapefruit, starfruit, strawberries, blackberries, raspberries, pineapple, and watermelon.

➤ Good sources of beta-carotene/vitamin A: apricots, cantaloupe, red and pink grapefruit and their juices, mangos, sapote, nectarines, loquats, persimmons, papayas, plantains, and prunes.

➤ Good sources of potassium: avocados, bananas, all melons, papayas, dried fruit, mangos, and oranges.

➤ Fruits that are especially high in fiber: berries, guavas, mangos, pears, plantains, pomegranates, rhubarb, and dried fruit.

➤ Good sources of vitamin E: mangos and avocados.

➤ Good sources of folate: watermelon, boysenberries, kiwi, oranges, plantains, strawberries, orange juice, grapefruit juice, and pineapple juice.

Shoppers Should Know

For peak sweetness and flavor, fruits should be eaten when they're ripe.

Colorful fruits add eye appeal, texture, flavor, and nutrients to any meal.

Fruits offer big flavor with modest amounts of calories. Most contain no fat and very little sodium.

Be careful not to bruise ripe fruit in the shopping basket or shopping bag.

Beta-carotene converts into an active form of vitamin A in the body. Cantaloupes, mangos, red grapefruit, and papaya are particularly rich in beta-carotene.

Ruby-red grapefruit has far more beta-carotene than white grapefruit.

Avocados are a high-fat fruit but the fat is monounsaturated, a heart-healthy type. Try thin slices of ripe avocado on sandwiches instead of mayonnaise.

Whole fruits have more fiber than fruit juices and no added sugar.

Freshly extracted juices have optimal flavor and nutrient value but are usually more expensive than fresh frozen or other forms of juice. Buy only pasteurized ciders. Fresh ciders can carry harmful bacteria.

Whole berries purchased economically in season can be frozen for year-round use.

Fresh fruit should be washed just before eating it. Store it covered but unwashed; it will keep longer.

Fresh fruit, packed in a plastic bag with a napkin, is an easy take-along sweet snack or part of a brown-bag lunch. Go beyond bananas, apples, and oranges; try grapes, cherries, and plums, for example.

Fruits and vegetables can provide all the vitamin C needed each day. In addition, when eaten together, vitamin C-rich foods triple the amount of iron absorbed from breads, grains, and cereals.

Citrus fruits include all varieties of oranges, grapefruits, tangerines, lemons, and limes.

Allow melons, apricots, plums, peaches, and pears to ripen at room temperature. Refrigerate ripe fruits, except for bananas, which should always be stored at room temperature.

When oranges and grapefruits are inexpensive or bags are on sale, squeezing fresh fruit for juice is more economical than buying juice.

Cantaloupes, honeydew, and other melons are easy to cube—and far less costly when purchased as whole or half melons than as cut fruit. The extra cost of cut, peeled fruit may be worthwhile for single servings or if you only need a little for a recipe.

Organically grown fruits and vegetables meet varying criteria based on state regulations. Certification standards are based on the length of time the soil has been kept free from pesticides, herbicides, and contaminants from nonorganic fields. Organic foods are processed, transported, and stored without artificial preservatives, colorings, or irradiation. Earth-friendly food production may yield better tasting fruit, but appearance and size of fruits and vegetables is less consistent and the price of organic fruit is often higher. Some supermarkets offer a wide variety of organic produce. Consumer demand and the philosophy of the store determines the amount, type, and pricing of organically grown produce.

Diets high in antioxidants (beta-carotene, vitamin E, vitamin C, and some phytochemicals) protect cells from damage. Diets high in antioxidants may reduce the incidence or severity of arthritis, coronary heart disease, cataracts, some neurological conditions, and cancers in some people.

Phytochemicals, food components that are not nutrients but provide health benefits, are present in many fruits. Several phytochemicals look promising based on limited studies. Ellegic acid, a phytochemical found in berries, may neutralize carcinogens before they can cause genetic changes in cells. Limonene, present in citrus fruit, may shrink tumors and prevent regrowth. It may also increase production of enzymes that may rid the body of carcinogens. Quercitin, found in grapes (and also wine from grapes), is a potent antioxidant that may protect cells from damage, aging, and environmental effects such as pollution. Terpenes, in oranges, seem to produce enzymes that may deactivate cancer-causing agents. Much research needs to be done before scientists agree on specific health benefits for specific phytochemicals. Most experts now agree that eating more fruits and vegetables promotes health and that most Americans should boost the intake of both fruits and vegetables.

Irradiated fruits carry a flower-like irradiation logo. Fruits and imported spices may be irradiated to destroy bacteria, and stay fresh longer. Some strawberries and other fruits are irradiated.

Frozen Fruit

Look For

- ➤ Frozen fruits packed without added sugar.
- ➤ Frozen 100 percent juice concentrate—single fruits or blends.
- ➤ Frozen fruit bars made with 100 percent fruit juice; chocolate-coated frozen bananas.
- ➤ Excellent sources of vitamin C: frozen strawberries and raspberries, and orange, tangerine, and grapefruit juices.
- ➤ Frozen cantaloupe balls, which contain beta-carotene/ vitamin A.

➤ Frozen strawberries, blackberries, boysenberries, and raspberries for fiber.

➤ Good sources of folate: frozen blackberries and strawberries, and orange, pineapple, and grapefruit juices.

Shoppers Should Know

Frozen fruit is comparable to fresh fruit in nutrient value.

Frozen 100 percent fruit juice concentrates are often the least expensive form of real 100 percent juice.

Frozen fruit-flavored juice beverage concentrates, punches, and drinks usually contain only 10 to 15 percent juice.

Frozen berries are usually less expensive than fresh. When thawed, they are somewhat mushy, but are fine for sauces or baking.

Frozen 100 percent lemon juice is similar to fresh-squeezed lemon juice in flavor.

"Homestyle" orange juices have some bits of fruit pulp, which makes them taste a bit more like fresh-squeezed juice but adds no useful amount of fiber.

Reduced-acid frozen orange juice is available for those who can not tolerate fresh or regular frozen orange juice.

Washed blueberries or stemmed, seedless grapes can be frozen on a baking sheet. Once frozen, transfer them to a freezer bag or airtight plastic container and use within a month. Keep them on hand for a refreshing snack that kids and adults enjoy, especially in warm weather.

Canned and Bottled Fruits and Juices

Look For

➤ Canned fruits packed in juice or light syrup.

➤ Juices and juice blends that are 100 percent juice.

➤ Jars of chilled orange segments, grapefruit segments, mango slices, papaya slices, pineapple chunks, and mixed fruit salads.

➤ Calcium-fortified juices—an excellent option, especially if intake of dairy products is limited.

➤ Sparkling apple cider or sparkling grape juice for festive occasions.

➤ Canned pumpkin and jars of stewed prunes. They are loaded with fiber, vitamins, and minerals.
➤ Applesauce, including varieties made with Granny Smith, McIntosh, and other apple varieties. Some are unsweetened.
➤ Reduced-sugar fruit pie fillings.
➤ Excellent sources of vitamin C: mandarin oranges, orange and grapefruit segments; orange, grapefruit, and tomato juices; cranberry juice cocktail and other vitamin C-fortified juices; and fortified fruit drinks.
➤ Good sources of beta-carotene/vitamin A: mandarin orange segments, sour cherries, apricots, apricot nectar, and tangerine juice.
➤ Juices that contain potassium: orange, grapefruit, tangerine, pineapple, and prune juices and tropical fruit blends.
➤ Pineapple juice is an excellent source of folate.

Shoppers Should Know
Fruit juices offer far more nutrition for the money than soft drinks.

Canned and bottled fruits are nutritious and convenient alternatives to fresh fruits, especially when a fruit is not in season.

When the label says 100 percent juice, it means the drink contains an unmodified pure juice with some fruit pulp. Fruit juices that are not 100 percent juice usually have color, taste, aroma, or other properties altered by additives or processing.

Single-serve juice boxes filled with 100 percent fruit juice and fruit cups are convenient and portable, but they are more expensive per serving than larger packages of juice and fruits.

Fruit packed in heavy syrup has more sugar than juice-packed fruits or fruits packed in light syrup. If fruit packed in heavy syrup is preferred, drain off the syrup to reduce calories from sugar.

A product labeled "no added sweeteners" has no added sugar, corn syrup, or artificial sweetener.

Bottled, canned, and frozen pure or blended juices made from concentrate, labeled 100 percent fruit juice, are nutritionally equivalent to fresh pressed juices but are less expensive.

A cup of orange juice made from frozen concentrate contains

two times the daily requirement for vitamin C.

Fortified juices contain vitamins or minerals added to boost the nutritional value. If you don't drink milk, juices with added calcium are a good choice.

Fruit drinks, punches, and juice beverages are sweetened water with a small amount of juice added. They don't count as a serving from the Fruit Group and fall within the Fats, Oils, and Sweets Group in the Food Guide Pyramid.

Full-strength cranberry juice is too acidic and concentrated to drink alone, so water and sweetener are added to make cranberry cocktails and cranberry-fruit blended drinks. Cranberry juice contains a substance that may prevent bladder infections in some people, so it might be helpful for those who are prone to urinary tract problems.

Apple and grape juices, apple cider, and pear and apricot nectars generally have less vitamin C than other fruit juices. Some have vitamins added; check the label.

Dry fruit-flavored drink mixes are available sweetened, unsweetened, or artificially sweetened. All are mixes of artificial flavor, colors, and additives, often with some vitamin C added.

Fruit-flavored sports drinks are mixes of water, artificial color, flavor, and additives with sugar, sodium and, sometimes, vitamins and minerals added.

Regular canned tomato and tomato-vegetable juice blends contain salt. Low-sodium tomato and vegetable juices are available for those on sodium-restricted diets.

Dried Fruits

Look For

> ➤ Dried prunes, including those flavored with orange or lemon essence. They are good sources of dietary fiber and vitamin A and are one of the least expensive dried fruits.
> ➤ Dried raisins, apricots, figs, peaches, pears, nectarines, bananas, cherries, currants, blueberries, sweetened cranberries (that look like raisins), and mango strips. All dried fruits are excellent sources of fiber and many provide potassium.

➤ Bags of chopped dried fruit to add to cereals, rice, and grains.
➤ Excellent sources of beta-carotene/vitamin A: dried apricots, mangos, nectarines, peaches, papayas, and prunes.
➤ Apricots and some other dried fruits, which absorb iron if they are dried on iron racks. Check the Nutrition Facts panel for iron levels of packaged dried fruits.

Shoppers Should Know

Dried fruits are shelf-stable and convenient. Look for them in the produce or baking supply sections of the store. Packaged dried fruits are labeled with a "use by" date.

Because water is extracted in drying fruits, all are concentrated sources of sugar and fiber. Small portions provide many key nutrients. Only 1 1/3 ounces (40 grams by weight) of a dried fruit is a standard serving. This is about 4 to 5 prunes or 2 tablespoons of raisins.

Some dried fruits are treated with sulfur dioxide to retain bright colors and moist texture. If sulfite is added, the label will say so. Individuals who are sensitive to sulfites should read labels carefully to avoid reactions, which can be severe.

Some dried fruits, including most bananas, cranberries, and diced dates have sugar added.

Banana chips are deep fried, often in tropical oil like coconut oil, and have sugar added. One ounce of dried banana chips has about 150 calories and nearly 10 grams of fat.

The yogurt coating on raisins is primarily sugar and hydrogenated palm kernel oil—about 135 calories and 6 grams of fat. Don't think of them as a source of low-fat, calcium-rich yogurt.

Dried shredded coconut is high in saturated fat but fine to use in small amounts for flavor and texture and as a garnish.

Only pitted prunes and dates should be given to young children. They can choke on prune or date pits.

Source: U.S. Department of Agriculture/U.S. Department of Health and Human Services, 1992.

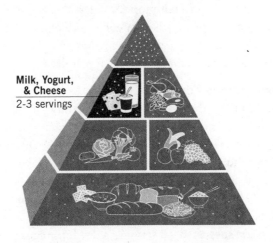

Milk, Yogurt, & Cheese in The Food Guide Pyramid

Milk, Yogurt, & Cheese
2-3 servings

• Fat (naturally occurring and added)   △ Sugars (added)

Milk and Milk Alternatives

Look For

➤ Fat-free and low-fat milks including fat-free milk, 1% fat milk, evaporated fat-free milk, nonfat dry milk, and nonfat or low-fat buttermilk for everyone over the age of 2.

➤ Reduced fat (2%) milk and reduced fat (2%) buttermilk, with fat content midway between fat-free and whole milk. They are good choices for young children, those who do not like fat-free milk, and individuals seeking to maintain weight.

➤ Whole milk for those who do not like low-fat milk or need to gain weight and for babies and toddlers who need some fat in milk for normal development.

➤ Nonfat or low-fat flavored milks such as chocolate milk.

➤ Fat-free or low-fat pasteurized eggnog.

➤ Low-fat sweetened condensed milk and canned, dry buttermilk for baking.

➤ Pasteurized goats milk for those intolerant of cows milk.

Soy or rice beverages for those who are vegetarians or cannot tolerate milk.
- Nonfat, 1%, 2% lactose-reduced, or lactase-treated milk for those who can not properly digest the lactose in milk.
- Sweet acidophilus milk for people with digestive problems.
- Hot cocoa mixes made with fat-free milk.

Shoppers Should Know

Milk and dairy products are the primary dietary sources of bone-building calcium. Milk also provides protein and minerals; almost all milk is fortified with vitamins A and D. Different milk and dairy products provide various amounts of fat, saturated fat, cholesterol, and calories.

One cup of milk equals 1 serving from the Milk Group in the Food Guide Pyramid. Two to three daily servings of low-fat dairy products are suggested—3 servings a day for pregnant women, teens, and young adults; and 4 servings daily for lactating women.

Milk is always labeled with a "sell by" date. The sell by date is the last date a food should be sold to allow several days of freshness for home use. Check date at the store and put milk in the refrigerator as soon as possible. Discard milk that has changed flavor, turned sour, or is curdled.

Milk can be stored in the freezer for up to 1 month. An "emergency quart" is a good idea especially if there are children or a pregnant woman in the household.

Nonfat dry milk and dry buttermilk are economical, nutritious choices to drink or use in cooking. They are shelf-stable; keep some on hand. Add dry milk powder to dishes to add calcium and other nutrients from milk.

Milk made from nonfat dry milk tastes better if it is chilled several hours before drinking or is mixed with a small amount of reduced fat (2%) milk.

Most milk sold in the United States is pasteurized, which means the micro-organisms that cause diseases (such as salmonella) and spoilage have been destroyed by heating, then quick-cooling.

Ultrapasteurization (also called ultra-high temperature

[UHT] processing) uses high heat (280°F for 2 to 4 seconds) and sterilized containers to destroy almost all bacteria in milk and cream. UHT dairy products can be stored unopened for up to 3 months without refrigeration. The heat processing significantly alters the flavor of the milk and/or cream.

Acidophilus milk has added "friendly bacteria" which can reintroduce helpful bacteria to the colon after diarrhea or antibiotic use.

Switching to a lower fat milk should be done gradually. Switch from whole milk (about 3.5% milkfat) to reduced fat (2% milkfat), then to low-fat (1% milkfat) or fat-free (0% milkfat). Let your palate adjust.

Buttermilk is made by culturing milk with helpful bacteria. Despite the name, it contains no butter. Salt is added for more flavor. When you want a creamy, thick texture and tangy taste, try low-fat or fat-free buttermilk. It is an excellent base for salad dressings and sauces, in cream soups, and in mashed potatoes. Buttermilk is higher in sodium than other milk.

Eggnog, sold around some holidays, is a blend of milk, eggs, sugar, cream, spices, and vanilla. Look for low-fat pasteurized eggnog.

Equal portions of low-fat (1%) milk and evaporated fat-free milk can replace light cream (half-and-half) in recipes.

Use evaporated fat-free milk or nonfat dry milk as a coffee creamer with a calcium bonus. Evaporated milk is concentrated milk fortified with vitamins A and D. Once opened, it needs refrigeration.

For coffee drinkers, a latte made with fat-free milk is an excellent choice. Each cup of latte contains about 1/2 cup of fat-free milk and about 150 milligrams of calcium.

Goats milk is easy to digest. It has slightly more fat than whole milk.

Chocolate milk made from low-fat and whole milk is available. Low-fat chocolate milk is made with fat-free milk, cocoa, thickening gums, artificial flavors, and sugar or sugar substitute. Chocolate milk made from whole milk usually contains similar ingredients plus sugar syrup. It is not a good choice for individuals with diabetes. Chocolate milk contains as much protein, calcium, and other nutrients as the milk it is made from. Check the label for calories and carbohydrate content.

Pasteurized chocolate drink contains some whey but no real milk. It provides only a bit of protein and calcium. It is sometimes found in the dairy case; bottled and canned chocolate drinks also can be found with the carbonated beverages.

Nondairy milk alternatives made from soy, almonds, or rice are usually low in fat and always cholesterol-free. Unless fortified, they do not provide the calcium and key nutrients of milk. A variety of plain and flavored soy and rice beverages are available. Check package label to compare nutrients.

Fat-free milk, soy milk, and rice beverages should not replace infant formula or milk for children under the age of 2. The fat and other nutrients in formula, whole, or reduced fat (2%) milk are necessary for brain and nerve development in infants and young children.

Bovine Somatotropin (BST) is an engineered hormone developed to increase milk production in cows. The milk from BST-treated cows can not be differentiated from milk from non-BST-treated cows according to the Food and Drug Administration.

Organic dairy products meet the requirements of the federal organic certification program. Livestock must be fed organically-produced feed, raised in a humane manner, and not be fed growth promoters, hormones, antibiotics, or other medications (other than vaccinations) on a regular basis. Organic dairy products must be processed separate from regular (non-organic) dairy products.

Yogurt and Yogurt Products

Look For

> Low-fat and nonfat (fat-free) yogurt and frozen yogurt with or without fruit flavoring, fruit topping, granola, or crunchy topping.
> Yogurts with active cultures. Most carry a label stating they meet National Yogurt Association criteria for live and active culture yogurt.

➤ Kefir and other low-fat yogurt drinks, with or without fruit flavor.

➤ Dairy-free fruited yogurt substitute for vegetarians.

Shoppers Should Know

One cup of yogurt is considered 1 serving from the Milk Group in the Food Guide Pyramid.

Eight ounces of plain yogurt has between 1 and 7 grams of fat depending on the type of milk used in making it. Low-fat varieties have less than 3 grams of fat. Nonfat yogurts are fat-free.

Yogurt is often thickened with milk solids and is an even better source of calcium than milk.

Yogurts with active cultures help keep your digestive system populated with helpful bacteria. After use of antibiotics, which destroy bacteria in the digestive tract, many are advised to eat yogurts with active cultures to restore good bacteria and normal elimination.

Some yogurts come in 8-ounce cartons; others come in 4- or 6-ounce containers. The nutrient values listed on the Nutrition Facts panel are for the full single-serving carton.

Yogurt should be stored in the refrigerator. If unopened, it should stay fresh up to 10 days after the "sell by" date.

Nonfat or low-fat yogurt is a good mayonnaise or sour cream replacement in some chilled foods. Mix some nonfat yogurt with mayonnaise or sour cream to create reduced-fat versions of homemade dips and spreads.

Custard-style yogurts are thicker but do not necessarily have more fat. Check the Nutrition Facts panel for fat content.

Most fruited and flavored yogurts are highly sweetened. Light yogurts contain sugar substitutes and are low-fat or fat-free. Reach for light yogurts if you're watching calories.

Chocolate-coated frozen yogurt bars have twice as many calories as uncoated bars and about 7 grams of fat instead of 1.

See additional comments on frozen yogurt in the Frozen Desserts section, page 91.

Cheese and Cheese Products

Look For

➤ Low-fat or part-skim cheeses including ricotta, part-skim mozzarella, scamorze, goat, string, feta, light cream cheese, Neufchâtel, and cottage cheese.

➤ Fat-free and low-fat cheese products containing 3 grams of fat or less per serving such as nonfat or low-fat cottage cheese, ricotta cheese, fromage blanc, and fat-free cream cheese.

➤ Any cheeses containing 5 grams of fat or less per serving including reduced-fat versions of your favorite cheeses.

➤ Light (reduced-fat), soft spreadable cheeses.

➤ Cheeses lower in sodium, or sodium-reduced cheeses if sodium is restricted, including some mozzarellas, ricotta, Jarlsberg, Neufchâtel, Swiss, Muenster, and cheddars. Check the Nutrition Facts panel.

Shoppers Should Know

One and a half ounces of natural cheese (such as cheddar), 2 ounces of processed cheese (such as American), or 1 1/2 cups of cottage cheese is considered a milk serving from the Food Guide Pyramid and the three choices provide similar amounts of calcium. These serving sizes are not the same as the amounts stated on the Nutrition Facts panel. Nutrients on the Nutrition Facts label are based on 1 ounce of most cheeses and 1/2 cup of cottage cheese.

Cheese should be stored in the refrigerator and sealed in the original packaging or well wrapped in foil or plastic wrap to keep it from drying out or absorbing odors from other foods. Packaged cheeses often have a "sell by" date; most cheese stays fresh at least one week after that date.

Cheese usually does not freeze well and changes texture if it is frozen.

Traditional cheeses, particularly high-fat ones, are major contributors to total fat and saturated fat in the diet. Many manufacturers have met consumer demand for reduced-fat and fat-free cheeses, but these products vary greatly in taste, texture, and cooking properties. Try some to find those you enjoy.

Fat-free sliced, shredded, and grated cheeses have a different texture and taste than cheese with fat. Use them when appropriate.

Use only small amounts of cheeses with 8 or more grams of fat per ounce (processed American, blue, brick, cheddar, Colby, fontina, Gruyère, and Havarti).

One pound (16 ounces) of hard or semi-firm cheese yields 4 to 5 cups of grated or shredded cheese.

Save money and fat calories and boost flavor by using small amounts of strong-flavored cheeses, such as Parmesan cheese, rather than large amounts of mild cheeses. Grated Parmesan has less than 2 grams of fat per tablespoon.

Creamed cottage cheese doesn't have as much cream (fat) as its name suggests. One-half cup of 1% fat creamed cottage cheese has 1 gram; 2% fat creamed cottage cheese has 2.5 grams; 4% creamed cottage cheese has 4.5 grams. Dry curd cottage cheese has 0.5 grams of fat.

Some brands of cottage cheese have extra calcium added, which is useful for those who don't drink milk.

Whole milk ricotta has 8 grams of fat in only 1/4 cup; part-skim ricotta has 5 to 6 grams. A fat-free version with no fat is available.

Unlike other cheeses that are rich in calcium and protein, cream cheese is primarily fat and contains little calcium and protein. Light and fat-free cream cheeses are available.

Processed cheeses are blends of different cheeses that are pasteurized to lengthen shelf life and treated with gelatin thickeners to give a smooth texture. They melt well.

Cheese spreads and cold pack cheese foods contain 3 to 9 grams of fat per serving and often a lot of sodium. Check the Nutrition Facts panel. Some brands are available in light forms. Only 2 tablespoons of cheese spread is a serving.

Breaded frozen cheese nuggets have 290 to 420 calories and 15 to 20 grams of fat per 3-ounce serving.

Puddings and Custards

Look For

> ➤ Rice, tapioca, and bread puddings, which have more grain and less sugar than butterscotch or chocolate puddings.
> ➤ Low-fat or fat-free prepared puddings, pudding mixes, and pudding pops.
> ➤ Low-fat or fat-free prepared custards or flans, or mixes.
> ➤ Pudding pops. They contain 70 to 80 calories without chocolate coating and 125 to 130 calories if coated.
> ➤ Chocolate mousse mixes that can be prepared with skim milk.
> ➤ Sugar-free mixes, if limiting calories or sugar.

Shoppers Should Know

A half cup is a standard serving of pudding or custard. Add raisins or other dried fruits to rice, bread, or tapioca pudding to boost fiber and nutrients. Prepare with fat-free or low-fat (1%) milk.

Sugar-free puddings, prepared from a mix with fat-free milk, contain 70 to 100 calories per 1/2-cup serving. Single-serve fat-free prepared pudding snacks have 100 calories per snack.

Chocolate lovers will find many types of chocolate pudding and chocolate blends in single serving puddings. Chocolate with a calcium bonus!

Single-serving fruit-flavored, chocolate, and vanilla snack puddings are made with fat-free milk but contain partially hydrogenated cottonseed oil. Some have artificial flavors and colors. Each 1/2-cup container provides 160 to 170 calories and 5 to 7 grams of fat including 2 grams of saturated fat.

Meat, Poultry, Fish, Dry Beans, Eggs, & Nuts in The Food Guide Pyramid

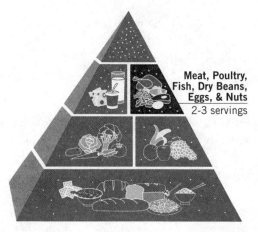

Meat, Poultry, Fish, Dry Beans, Eggs, & Nuts
2-3 servings

• Fat (naturally occurring and added)   Δ Sugars (added)

Beef, Pork, Lamb, Veal, and Game Meats

Look For

➤ Meats labeled extra-lean. They have less than 5 grams of fat, less than 2 grams of saturated fat, and less than 95 milligrams of cholesterol per 3 1/2-ounce cooked serving. All are excellent choices.

➤ Meats labeled lean. They have less than 10 grams of fat, less than 4 1/2 grams of saturated fat, and less than 95 milligrams of cholesterol per 3 1/2-ounce cooked serving.

➤ Meat graded USDA Select or Choice.

➤ The leanest cuts of well-trimmed beef including flank, sirloin, and tenderloin; round, ribeye, T-bone, porterhouse, and cubed steaks; and eye of round roast, rib, chuck, and rump roasts.

➤ The leanest cuts of well-trimmed pork including fresh, canned, cured, and boiled ham; Canadian bacon; and pork tenderloin, loin chops, rib chops, and roasts.

➤ Lean, well-trimmed cuts of lamb and veal including lamb

roast, chops, and leg; and veal chops, arm steaks, blade steaks, "scallopini" cuts, cutlets, and roasts.

➤ Game that is lean including venison, antelope, beaver, rabbit, beefalo, bison, buffalo, caribou, elk, and goat.

➤ Lean or extra-lean ground beef, pork, lamb, and veal (at least 90 percent lean). Check the "sell-by" date; ground meats are especially perishable.

Shoppers Should Know

Meats are good sources of protein, highly absorbable iron and zinc, vitamin B12, niacin, potassium, phosphorus, and other minerals. Meat also provides fat, saturated fat, and cholesterol—substances best limited to moderate amounts.

The Food Guide Pyramid recommends 5 to 7 ounces of meat or its equivalent from the Meat Group each day.

One serving of meat from the Food Guide Pyramid is only 2 to 3 ounces of cooked lean meat, poultry, or fish. Three ounces of cooked meat is about the size of a deck of cards, an audiocassette, or the size of the palm of a woman's hand.

One pound of boneless lean meat should yield about 4 (3-ounce) servings when cooked.

If you cook whole steaks, limit portion size by thinly slicing the cooked meat and fanning it out. A moderate serving will look like a more generous portion.

If you want to serve a meat portion larger than 3 ounces, plan on 2 standard servings (6 ounces cooked) and don't eat servings from the meat group at other meals that day.

Always check the "sell-by" date on fresh meats. Cook whole and cut fresh meats within 3 to 5 days of purchase (or the "sell-by" date) and ground meat within 1 to 2 days or wrap and freeze it for later use.

Refrigerate or freeze fresh meat immediately. Store it in the coldest part of the refrigerator. To maintain quality longer, wrap it in freezer paper, freezer bags, or plastic film before freezing it. Mark the wrapper with contents and date frozen.

Trimming visible fat can cut the fat content considerably.

Barbecuing, broiling, grilling, and roasting are cooking methods that drain fat.

For ground beef, ground round is usually the leanest followed by ground sirloin, ground chuck, and then regular ground beef. If you don't see ground round, the meat cutter can usually grind it from round steak. Ground sirloin is usually more expensive than ground round but many prefer the flavor of ground sirloin for burgers. A less expensive ground beef, cooked and drained, will taste about the same when cooked in sauce or combined with highly flavored ingredients.

Ground meats should be cooked to at least medium doneness (at least 160°F) for food safety. Never serve ground meat raw or rare. Steak tartare and rare burgers are risky.

When cooking ground meats, drain fat well before combining cooked ground meat with other ingredients.

Meat graded Select has less fat but is less tender and flavorful than meat graded Choice. Prime grade meats contain the most marbling (internal fat), are most costly and tender, and are primarily sold to fine restaurants.

The color of a meat indicates freshness. Beef should be bright red with no grayish areas. Both young veal and pork are pale grayish pink. Older veal and pork are darker pink. Lamb varies in color depending on what it was fed.

Higher-fat meats include pork spareribs, beef ribs, short ribs, tongue, ground pork, most sausages, and bacon.

Organ meats, such as beef liver, kidney, and heart, are very high in iron and many vitamins but also high in cholesterol.

Veal is lower in total fat than most other red meats but is higher in cholesterol—usually 90 to 130 milligrams of cholesterol and 130 to 170 calories per 3-ounces of veal in comparison to 70 to 85 milligrams cholesterol and 150 to 250 calories per 3-ounce serving of beef.

Some high-fat meats, such as corned beef brisket, are available in low-fat forms from processors that choose the leanest cuts and trim them very well. These meats are usually branded and say "lean" or "extra lean" on the front label. Check the label for sodium content if sodium is a concern.

When pork is cured to make ham, salt is added. Although most ham is now lean, it is usually high in sodium.

Preseasoned and precooked roasts, ribs, and other meats save time but cost considerably more than fresh, raw meats. Check the sodium level.

Beef certified by the USDA as natural has been grown without hormones, antibiotics, or preservatives. It carries a premium price.

Cured meats are processed with salt, sugar, and often nitrites to preserve them and add flavor. Ham, bacon, some sausages, and lunch meats are cured. The USDA regulates the amount of nitrite used in curing meats and requires the addition of vitamin C, sodium ascorbate, or sodium erythorbate to bind the added nitrites because nitrites have been associated with increased risk of cancer in some studies.

Canned hams are fully cooked. Fresh ham labeled "smoked" or "aged" does not mean that the meat has been cooked. Unless the label says "fully cooked," cook ham like fresh pork.

Avoid buying meat in a package that is not tightly sealed, contains excessive juices or is not cold. Do not buy meat having any brownish or grayish patches.

Always defrost and marinate meat in the refrigerator. Do not use the marinade as a sauce unless it is first brought to a rolling boil.

Poultry and Game Birds

Look For

- ➤ All types of poultry, including chicken, turkey, Cornish game hens, duck, pheasant, squab, and quail.
- ➤ Plenty of chicken and turkey. Watch for sales and stock up when prices are low.
- ➤ Table-ready rotisserie or roasted chicken, turkey breast, and breast tenderloin.
- ➤ Lean or extra-lean ground turkey and chicken. Check the label for fat content.
- ➤ Game birds that are extra-lean including guinea fowl, pheasant, quail, emu, and ostrich.
- ➤ Game birds that are lean such as squab and skinless duckling.
- ➤ Canned chicken packed in broth or water.

Shoppers Should Know

White meat of poultry (the breast) has less fat than dark meat (thighs or legs).

Half of the calories in chicken are in the skin. Buy skinless parts or remove the skin of cooked poultry before eating it. Skinless chicken has the same fat content whether it is cooked with or without skin, and cooking chicken with skin on retains moisture.

Skinless, boneless chicken breasts usually command premium prices. Watch for sales or buy chicken breasts with the bone in. Remove skin before eating.

Chicken and turkey wings have a high percentage of skin and are higher in fat than other parts of the birds.

Whole or split broiler-fryer chickens (3 to 4 pounds) are usually less expensive than chicken parts. Save money by cutting up whole chickens and packing similar parts in freezer wrap or bags for use in different meals.

Ground poultry is very perishable. Cook it within 1 or 2 days or freeze it.

Ground turkey breast or chicken breast is generally lower in fat than regular ground turkey or chicken (or nuggets or rolls), which usually contains skin and dark meat.

Chicken livers are very rich in vitamins and minerals but high in cholesterol. Check the "sell-by" date and cook chicken livers within 2 days of purchase.

Frozen turkey and rock Cornish hens are often less expensive than fresh.

Turkey parts, often thighs, are economical and healthy choices. Roast the thigh and serve it sliced or diced in salads. Barbecue turkey legs or use them to make soup.

Seasoned, marinated, or precooked chicken and turkey breasts or parts save time but command premium prices.

Self-basting turkeys are injected with fat and are higher in fat than fresh turkeys. They also may be seasoned with salt, making them higher in sodium.

Rotisserie chicken tends to be high in sodium. Removing the skin of rotisserie chicken before eating it removes much of the sodium and fat.

Up and Down the Aisles

Use fresh poultry within 2 days of purchase or freeze it. Frozen poultry should thaw in the refrigerator, never at room temperature. A frozen turkey can take up to 4 days to thaw.

For food safety, poultry should be rinsed under cold water and cooked thoroughly. Use a separate cutting board for raw poultry. Wash the board and utensils with hot, soapy water and rinse with a chlorine bleach solution (2 teaspoons chlorine bleach mixed with 1 quart of water) after each contact with raw poultry. Do not cut vegetables or other foods you will eat without cooking on the same board that has been used for raw poultry.

Cook prestuffed chickens within 1 day after purchase. They are very perishable and do not freeze well.

Organically raised poultry is raised in accordance with federal standards for the organic production of farm animals and is fed organically produced feed and raised in a humane manner. Growth-promoting hormones and antibiotics (given in the absence of illness) are prohibited.

Free-range chickens are no more nutritious than traditional chickens and are more likely to carry bacteria because their feed does not contain additives that control bacterial growth. Some people believe free-range chickens have more flavor.

Duck is leaner than it used to be. Cooking it so the skin is very crisp or removing the skin makes duck a good choice. Duck and pheasant, well-drained and eaten without skin, are similar in fat content to chicken and turkey.

Fish and Seafood

Look For

> ➤ A seafood department with a fresh, mildly seaweedy, but not strong, fishy smell.
> ➤ Seafood that has been kept well-iced or frozen. Cooked fish products should be separated from raw seafood.
> ➤ Ways to eat at least 2 servings a week of fish and seafood.
> ➤ Fresh finfish that is moist and firm with bright eyes, red gills, firm, moist flesh, scales that cling tightly to the skin, and no fishy smell. There should be no browning or drying around the edges of filleted fish.
> ➤ Fresh shrimp with firm meat, mild odor, and natural pale

gray color that are not slippery or slimy. They should have no black or dry spots. Cooked shrimp should have reddish shells, firm pale pink meat, and a pleasant odor. Check the seafood and deli departments, salad bar, frozen food case, and canned fish aisle for seafood choices.

➤ Lobster, crab, and crayfish, sold live unless they are frozen, canned, or cooked. Shucked (with shells removed) oysters and scallops should have a mild, fresh scent and somewhat clear (not milky or slimy) liquid.

➤ Surimi—imitation crab, scallops, lobster, and shrimp.

➤ Canned fish with soft edible bones, such as sardines and salmon, for calcium. Both are also high in omega-3 fatty acids.

➤ Fresh fish, frozen fish without breading, and canned fish packed in water or broth, which are lower in fat and calories than breaded or oil-packed fish.

➤ Fresh and salt-free canned fish, if on sodium-restricted diets.

➤ Frozen, farm-raised, or locally caught fish, which are usually less expensive than fresh fish that has been flown in.

➤ Easy-to-prepare, cleaned shrimp, scallops, mussels, octopus, calamari, or mixed seafoods in the frozen foods case.

➤ Reputable shellfish dealers who buy from harvesters licensed with the National Shellfish Sanitation Program (NSSP).

Shoppers Should Know

Two and a half to 3 ounces of cooked fish or other seafood equals 1 serving from the Meat Group in the Food Guide Pyramid. (Weight includes edible seafood without shells, skin, bones, etc.) Plan on buying 3/4 pound per serving of whole fish; 1/2 pound per serving of dressed fish or fish with bones; 1/4 to 1/3 pound per person of fish fillets, scallops, peeled shrimp, cooked shelled lobster, or crabmeat.

Salmon, tuna, mackerel, rainbow trout, bluefish, herring, bonito, pompano, sardines, and anchovies, are good sources of heart-healthy omega-3 fatty acids.

Omega-3 fatty acids, found especially in higher-fat fish, have been shown to protect against heart disease by thinning the blood, lowering blood fats, and decreasing the tendency toward plaque formation, which narrows arteries.

All fish and shellfish (crustaceans, mollusks, and cephalopods) are good sources of protein, vitamins, and minerals. They are low in saturated fat and lower in total fat and calories than most other sources of protein.

Crustaceans, including shrimp, crayfish, and lobster, are higher in cholesterol than other seafood but very low in saturated fat and total fat. Scallops and mussels are low in fat, saturated fat, and cholesterol. Prepare and serve them in ways that do not add a lot of fat.

Oysters, clams, scallops, and mussels are mollusks.

Octopus and squid are cephalopods, a shellfish that carries its shell inside. Cleaned and dressed octopus and squid are available fresh or frozen and are particularly popular in Greek, Italian, Asian, and Portuguese cooking.

Whole fish and dressed fish (with head, tail, and fins removed) cost less than steaks and fillets but you need to buy more because there is some waste.

Aquaculture is the cultivation of farm-raised seafoods in ponds, cages, tanks, or pens attached to natural bodies of water. This method allows control of the water supply and increases seafood yield usually reducing fishing costs and prices to consumers. Farm-raised catfish and salmon are less expensive than fish from natural lakes and streams but are not as flavorful.

Whole salmon and salmon steaks are usually less costly than salmon fillets. Canned pink salmon is less expensive than red sockeye salmon.

Surimi is imitation shellfish made from processing and molding mild-flavored fish and adding color and flavor so that it looks like crab, scallops, lobster, or shrimp. It is lower in price and cholesterol, but higher in sodium than fresh seafood.

Drain oil from canned tuna and sardines or buy water-packed tuna. Canned chunk light tuna costs less than solid white tuna and is equally healthful.

Shrimp is sold in many sizes. Larger sizes are more expensive. Per pound there are fewer than 15 colossal shrimp; 31 to 35 large shrimp; and over 70 tiny shrimp.

Fresh fish and shellfish should be kept tightly wrapped in the coldest part of the refrigerator. Use it within 1 to 2 days of purchase. Rinse all seafood with cold water before cooking it.

Thaw frozen fish in the refrigerator and use thawed fish within 24 hours.

For food safety reasons, eating raw shellfish, mollusks, and fish (sushi and sashimi) should be avoided.

Seviche is raw fish or shellfish marinated in lime juice or other acid. Although the fish turns firm and opaque, it carries the same health risks as other raw seafood.

Breading and frying seafood (or any food) raises fat, calorie, and sodium levels. Frozen batter-dipped or breaded fish, shrimp, and scallops are high in fat.

Smoked salmon (lox) and other smoked fish may be low in fat but are high in sodium.

Cocktail sauce is a fat-free condiment for seafood. Tartar sauce, however, is usually high in fat.

Packaged Meats/Cold Cuts

Look For

- ➤ Lean sliced meats, such as plain or seasoned lean roast beef, turkey, and lean ham.
- ➤ Processed luncheon meats and sausages labeled fat-free or low-fat.
- ➤ Canadian-style bacon, turkey salami, and turkey ham. Most brands are low-fat—check the Nutrition Facts panel.
- ➤ Fat-free or reduced-fat hot dogs, sausages, cold cuts, and breakfast meats.
- ➤ Gourmet poultry sausages with herbs, fruits, and nuts.
- ➤ Freshness dates on packages—usually a "sell-by" date. Packaged meats stay fresh longer than most other meats, at least 1 week after the "sell-by" date, if tightly sealed.
- ➤ Plain roast beef, turkey, or chicken breast or reduced-sodium varieties of cold cuts and sausages if sodium is restricted.

Shoppers Should Know

It's smart to compare the Nutrition Facts panel on packaged luncheon meats.

Most regular sausage products, including hot dogs and cold cuts, are high in sodium and fat.

Processed meats, sausages, and luncheon meats can contain large quantities of hidden fat, saturated fat, and sodium. Many reduced-fat varieties are now available. Lean deli meats are convenient and add variety and flavor without a lot of fat.

Turkey and chicken franks do not always have less fat or calories than beef or beef and pork franks. Check the Nutrition Facts panel.

Canadian bacon is much lower in fat than regular bacon. Turkey bacon varies in fat content. Check the Nutrition Facts panel.

Liverwurst and other sausages containing liver and specialty sausages containing organ meats are high in cholesterol and fat but rich in iron, vitamins, and minerals. Eat them only occasionally, or choose reduced-fat versions.

Legumes

Legumes can be counted as servings from either the Meat Group or the Vegetable Group on the Food Guide Pyramid, but not both.

Look For

> ➤ Split peas, black-eyed peas, kidney beans, navy beans, black beans, adzuki beans, great Northern beans, lentils, garbanzos (chickpeas), lima beans, pinto beans, and varieties of heirloom beans. Look for dried beans with smooth surfaces and bright colors, with no holes or discolorations in bags that aren't torn. All are excellent sources of protein, fiber, iron, folate, and zinc.
> ➤ Tofu (soybean curd), which is a high-protein, cholesterol-free meat substitute. It is usually found in the produce section. Check the freshness date on the wrapper. Buy tofu that has been processed with calcium to boost your calcium intake.
> ➤ Soy products such as tofu, tempeh, miso, soy burgers (veg-

gie burgers), and vegetarian sausages.

➤ Canned legumes including reduced-fat or fat-free vegetarian baked and refried beans.

➤ Hummus, a spread made from garbanzo beans (chickpeas).

Shoppers Should Know

Legumes are plants that produce pods with edible seeds—beans, peas, and lentils.

A half cup of cooked peas, lentils, or beans or 3 ounces of tofu is equal in portion size to 1 ounce of meat.

Peas, lentils, and beans add protein, minerals, and variety to meatless meals. They add thickness and heartiness to soups, chilis, stews, and casseroles.

Dry split peas and lentils, an inexpensive meat substitute, join eggs as the least expensive source of protein. One pound, about 2 1/2 cups of dry beans or lentils, swells to 5 to 6 cups when cooked. Most dried beans take about 1 1/2 hours to cook; lentils cook in 30 to 45 minutes.

Canned and frozen beans save time. Most canned beans have added salt. Rinse canned beans under cold running water if sodium is restricted.

Organically grown beans are certified to be produced in accordance with federal organic certification guidelines using methods to enhance soil fertility, biologic cycles, and diversity. No prohibited fertilizers or other chemicals have been applied to the soil for at least 3 years prior to marketing as organic.

Blended bean mixes and gourmet packs of beans are usually at least three times as expensive as plain legumes.

The fiber found in lentils and beans may help lower blood cholesterol and reduce the risk of some types of cancer.

Peanuts are actually legumes—not nuts. Since most people would look for information about peanuts in the section on nuts, we describe peanut products on page 82.

Dried beans and peas can produce gas and bloating in the digestive tract, especially if they aren't eaten often. Legumes that are usually easier to digest include adzuki beans, anasazi beans, black-eyed peas, lentils, mung beans, tofu, and tempeh.

Soy promotes estrogen production in women and may help

protect against heart disease. Soy products contain several phytochemicals including genestein and flavenoids that have been shown to keep cancer-causing agents from attaching to cells and prevent growth of tumors.

Miso, a fermented soybean paste, can be used to season foods and in salad dressings.

Soybeans are high in iron but contain several inhibitors that block some iron absorption. Traditional methods used to produce fermentation in soy foods (tempeh, miso, soy sauce, tofu) increase the availability of iron by breaking down these inhibitors, making fermented soy foods a useful source of iron.

Soft, "silken" tofu is lighter and more delicate than regular tofu. It can be blended with fruit into beverages or seasoned and used as a dip or spread. Add sliced, firm tofu to soups, stir-fries, and vegetables.

Textured vegetable protein (TVP) is made by removing 90 percent of the carbohydrate from defatted soy flour. The result is a concentrated protein sold as granules or chunks to be used as a meat replacement that contains no fat or cholesterol.

Products that contain soy may list "textured vegetable protein," "hydrolyzed vegetable protein," "soy protein," or "soy concentrate" on the ingredient panel.

Meat substitutes made from soy such as burgers, hot dogs, or breakfast sausages strive for a meaty flavor and texture. Some brands fare better than others in taste tests.

Some legume and soy-based convenience foods have a lot of fat. Meatless does not necessarily equal low-fat. Check the Nutrition Facts panel.

Eggs and Egg Substitutes

Look For
> ➤ Fresh, uncracked clean eggs kept in a refrigerated case. Open the container to check.
> ➤ The USDA inspection shield on grade AA and A eggs. Inspection ensures proper quality and dating, and that eggs have been kept refrigerated before and after packing.
> ➤ Egg substitutes, if you are restricting cholesterol or want to use raw eggs in a recipe (such as Caesar salad). Because

they are pasteurized, they are safe to eat even if uncooked.
➤ Tiny quail eggs to use as garnishes and in gourmet cooking.

Shoppers Should Know

If there is a price difference of 7 cents or less per dozen between two sizes of eggs, the larger eggs are a better buy. Eggs come in six sizes—jumbo, extra-large, large, medium, small, and pee-wee. Most stores offer three sizes.

One egg is equal in protein to 1 ounce of meat.

Eggs are an economical, excellent source of protein and contain almost all essential vitamins and minerals. They are quick to fix and versatile.

One large egg contains 6 grams of protein, 5 grams of fat (3 grams of unsaturated fat, 2 grams of saturated fat), 210 milligrams of cholesterol, and 70 calories.

All of the cholesterol and fat is in the yolk of the egg. The American Heart Association advises no more than 4 egg yolks per week per person. Use egg substitutes or egg whites in place of more eggs.

Some branded eggs come from chickens fed special feed. These eggs are rich in vitamin E (25 percent of the Daily Value per egg) and some research suggests that they do not raise serum cholesterol levels.

To reduce cholesterol and fat, 2 egg whites can replace 1 whole egg in many recipes; 2 egg whites plus 1 egg can replace 2 eggs. Most baking recipes use large eggs.

Brown eggs, fertile eggs, and nest eggs are equal in nutrient value to white eggs.

Eggs will keep up to 4 weeks in the refrigerator at 40°F or below.

Egg substitutes vary in ingredients. Some have fat and others do not. Most are sold frozen in small cartons. Generally 1/4 cup egg substitute equals 1 fresh egg. Egg substitutes cost about twice as much as fresh eggs.

For food safety reasons (potential salmonella), soft-cooked or raw eggs in beverages, uncooked meringues, homemade ice creams, and salad dressings should be avoided.

Canned, dried, pasteurized egg whites are sometimes available in the baking supply aisle of the store.

The egg industry is testing ways to pasteurize eggs in the shell to reduce risk of salmonella. Pasteurized whole eggs (removed from shells) are available to food service operators but are now becoming available in supermarkets. Watch for both forms of pasteurized eggs.

Commercial vegetarian egg substitutes are made from potato starch, tapioca flour, leavening agents, and a vegetable-derived gum.

When storing eggs, keep them in the original carton to maintain freshness.

Nuts and Seeds/Nut Butters

Look For

- ➤ Unsalted nuts in the baking supply aisle; salted nuts with snack foods; whole nuts in shells with produce.
- ➤ Nuts that are firm, with smooth surfaces and uniform color.
- ➤ Nut butters, especially reduced-fat varieties.
- ➤ Reduced-fat and regular peanut butter. Two tablespoons of either contain 120 to 150 milligrams of sodium, which is not excessive unless sodium is restricted. If sodium is a concern, choose unsalted peanut butter.
- ➤ Chestnuts, the only low-fat nut.
- ➤ Oil-on-top or "natural" nut butters for less saturated fat.
- ➤ Tahini, sesame butter, whole sesame seeds, almonds, and almond butter—all of which contain some calcium.

Shoppers Should Know

Two tablespoons of peanut butter is a standard serving equal to 1 ounce of meat. But this much peanut butter provides about 190 calories, the caloric equivalent of about 3 ounces of lean meat.

Smooth, chunky, and crunchy-style peanut butters are nutritionally equal—some are just ground more finely.

Regular peanut butter contains about 17 grams of fat per 2 tablespoon serving and 190 calories; reduced-fat peanut butter contains 12 grams of fat per 2 tablespoon serving and 180 to 200 calories. Reduced-fat peanut butter usually has added sugar.

Seeds, nuts, and seed and nut butters provide protein, fiber, and antioxidant vitamin E but are high in fat and calories. Seeds and nuts contain unsaturated fats, which are more heart-healthy than fats found in meat and dairy products.

The fat in most nuts—almonds, cashews, chestnuts, filberts, pistachios, macadamia, peanuts, and pecans—is primarily monounsaturated, like that found in olive oil.

The fat in walnuts, Brazil nuts, pine nuts, and sesame, sunflower, and pumpkin seeds is primarily polyunsaturated, like that found in corn oil.

One ounce of shelled nuts contains 160 to 195 calories and 13 to 22 grams of fat.

Macadamia nuts have the most fat (21 grams per ounce) followed by filberts (hazelnuts), Brazil nuts, pecans, and walnuts.

Dry-roasted nuts have about the same calories and fat as oil-roasted nuts.

Coconut is a source of saturated fat, but a few shreds of coconut as a garnish contribute flavor and texture and little total or saturated fat.

Cashews, peanuts, and almonds have a bit less fat than walnuts and pecans. Almonds provide some calcium.

One ounce of shelled nuts contains as much fiber as two slices of whole-wheat bread.

Sesame butter is a peanut butter-like spread made from whole ground sesame seeds. Tahini is a thinner, milder version made from hulled sesame seeds.

Hydrogenating some of the oil in peanut butter keeps the oil from separating but increases the saturated fat content a bit.

Sometimes sugar is added to peanut butter to balance and improve the flavor, especially in reduced-fat peanut butter. There is no real advantage to sugar-free peanut butter.

Once opened, large containers of peanut butter should be refrigerated. Keep a small amount at room temperature. You'll use less if it's easy to spread.

Nuts should be refrigerated or stored frozen in an airtight container unless they are vacuum-packed. Unopened vacuum-packed nuts can be stored at room temperature in your pantry.

Toasting nuts a few minutes intensifies their flavor. You can then use fewer nuts in recipes or toppings.

Flaxseed, which can be used in breads or sprinkled on salads, is rich in omega-3 fatty acids.

Fats, Oils, and Sweets in The Food Guide Pyramid

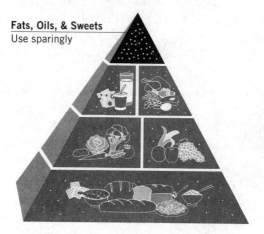

Fats, Oils, & Sweets
Use sparingly

Source: U.S. Department of Agriculture/U.S. Department of Health and Human Services, 1992.

• Fat (naturally occurring and added)   Δ Sugars (added)

Butter, Margarine, and Spreads

Look For

> ➤ Soft tub margarines or spreads or squeezable bottles or sprays. The first ingredient on the label should be liquid vegetable oil or water.
> ➤ Low-fat, light, reduced-calorie, or diet margarines and spreads.
> ➤ Butter substitutes (sprinkles or sprays) for seasoning vegetables and popcorn. They are fat- and cholesterol-free.
> ➤ Fat-free spreads in sticks or tubs. See if they pass your taste test.
> ➤ Margarines with added buttermilk or yogurt solids, or margarine-butter blends. They offer some of the health

benefits of margarine with more of the flavor of butter.
➤ Butter, to be used in moderation.
➤ Unsalted butter or margarine, if sodium is restricted.

Shoppers Should Know

Regular butter and margarine have 100 to 110 calories per tablespoon; spreadables have about 80 calories; whipped varieties have about 70 calories; light varieties have 50 to 60 calories.

Both butter and margarine are at least 80 percent fat and have 12 grams of fat per tablespoon.

Butter provides 11 milligrams of cholesterol per tablespoon; margarine has none.

Salted butter keeps longer; unsalted (sweet) butter has a more delicate flavor. Keep one stick in the refrigerator, the rest in the freezer.

Unsalted (sweet) butter contains less than 20 milligrams of sodium per tablespoon; regular salted butter has about 110 to 120 milligrams of sodium per tablespoon.

Many people find that butter melts better, works better in baked goods, and tastes better than margarine.

Margarines are mixtures of water or milk and hydrogenated vegetable oil.

Trans-fatty acids in hydrogenated and partially hydrogenated fats (such as stick margarine) have been shown to increase levels of LDL "bad" cholesterol in the blood and may decrease levels of HDL "good" cholesterol.

Soft, spreadable margarines are more heart-healthy than stick margarines or butter. They are less hydrogenated.

Whipped butter has air whipped in. It has fewer calories and less fat than stick butter and spreads well.

Light or whipped butter and margarines are not recommended for baking or frying. Their added water causes spattering and poor baking results.

Light butter with 6 grams of fat and 50 calories per tablespoon is made from butter and skim milk with added ingredients. Nondairy additives add color and flavor.

Granulated butter substitutes work best on hot, moist foods such as vegetables. They add flavor without fat. Flavored butter granules are also available.

Butter-flavored sprays can be used liberally because they are fat-free. Try butter-flavored spray between layers of phyllo dough or for other cooking uses to replace melted butter.

Cooking Fats

Look For

➤ Butter and margarine to use in moderation and for selected uses. See page 85.

➤ No-stick cooking sprays, including olive oil, garlic, and butter-flavored varieties.

Shoppers Should Know

Use the Nutrition Facts panel to help you choose cooking fats lower in total fat, saturated fat, and cholesterol. See the next page for information on vegetable oils.

All fats should be used sparingly in cooking and at the table.

Many recipes work perfectly well using less butter or other fat than specified. Reduce cooking fat to the lowest level that still yields tasty results.

Applesauce, prune purée, or mashed ripe bananas can be substituted for up to half the fat in many recipes for cakes, muffins, and quick breads.

Using no-stick cooking sprays reduces the need for oil to keep food from sticking to skillets and pans. Nonaerosol pump sprays are environmentally friendly.

Chicken fat contains primarily heart-healthy monounsaturated fat (the type found in olive oil) and only 10 milligrams of cholesterol per tablespoon. Each tablespoon has 13 grams of fat including 4 grams of saturated fat and 120 calories.

Lard and butter are primarily saturated fat. Use them in moderation and substitute heart-healthy fats whenever possible.

The most popular all-vegetable shortening has 12 grams of fat and 110 calories per tablespoon. Although the label indicates 4 grams of monounsaturated fat (and 50 percent less saturated fat than butter), the first ingredient listed is partially hydrogenated oil. It may be a monounsaturated fat but it acts more like saturated fat in the body because it is partially hydrogenated.

Hot oil or shortening shouldn't be poured into shortening

containers unless the container is metal. Most brands now come in paper "cans."

Vegetable Oils

Look For
> ➤ Olive, almond, canola, rapeseed, avocado, and peanut oils. All contain primarily monounsaturated fat.
> ➤ Safflower, sunflower, corn, flaxseed, walnut, sesame, and soybean oils. All contain primarily polyunsaturated fat.
> ➤ Small bottles of sesame, avocado, and nut oils.
> ➤ Infused oils flavored with garlic, herbs, lemon, or other seasonings.
> ➤ Cold-pressed, unrefined oils.

Shoppers Should Know
All oils and fats are high in calories (about 120 calories per tablespoon) and fat and should be used in moderation.

Most liquid oils are less saturated and, therefore, more heart-healthy than solid fats.

Polyunsaturated oils (corn, sunflower, and safflower), labeled "cold-pressed," are unrefined oils. More sensitive to heat and light, they should be refrigerated. They carry more protective antioxidant vitamin E and essential fatty acids than the same oils that are regularly processed. Cold-pressed oils usually carry a premium price. Some studies suggest that cold-pressed oils contain other protective substances but more research is needed to validate that benefit.

Small amounts of flavored and nut oils—sesame, walnut, almond, chili, garlic, mushroom, etc.—add great flavor to foods. Keep them refrigerated; they are more perishable than other bottled oils.

Some oils are lighter in color and milder in flavor than similar oils. They may say "light" on the label but usually do not contain less calories or fat than regular oils. This use of the word "light" describes a color or characteristic and is the exception to the reduced-fat and calorie regulation.

Extra-virgin olive oil comes from the first pressing of the olives. It is more expensive and flavorful than other grades of olive oil and it changes flavor when heated to high temperatures. Use it in dishes in which you can appreciate its flavor. If a dish calls for high heat, lots of spices, or strong flavors, virgin olive oil—or a lesser grade—is adequate.

Coconut, palm, and palm kernel oils (sometimes called tropical oils) are very high in saturated fat. Most people don't cook with coconut oil (except ethnic dishes), but tropical oils are used in processed foods, so watch for them on ingredient lists.

Salad Dressings

Look For

➤ Fat-free or low-fat salad dressings.

➤ Light or reduced-fat salad dressings.

➤ Reduced-fat, light, or fat-free mayonnaise and sandwich spreads.

Shoppers Should Know

Two tablespoons is a standard serving of salad dressing, but many people use more, especially on large salads.

Regular dressings contain 10 to 20 grams of fat in a 2-tablespoon serving; reduced-fat and light dressings have 1 to 7 grams of fat; low-fat dressings have 3 grams or less of fat per 2-tablespoon serving; fat-free dressings have 0.5 grams of fat or less per 2-tablespoon serving and 5 to 20 calories per tablespoon. Check the Nutrition Facts Panel.

Vegetable oil in salad dressing doesn't contain cholesterol but oil is 100 percent fat. It may say cholesterol-free, but it has fat and calories.

Generally, oil-and-vinegar-type dressings have less fat per tablespoon than creamy, cheese, or ranch-type dressings. Check the Nutrition Facts panel for fat content of your favorite brands.

Fat-free does not mean calorie-free. Many fat-free dressings have calories from sugar, starch, or thickeners. Individuals with diabetes should carefully check the carbohydrate content of fat-free and reduced-calorie dressings.

To reduce fat and calories, use lower-calorie dressings or smaller amounts of regular dressings.

Thick dressings (like blue cheese dressing) can be thinned

with plain low-fat yogurt, milk, buttermilk, broth, fruit juice, or water to reduce calories per serving. You also will use less because it takes less thinned dressing to coat greens.

Low-calorie dressings make great marinades for meat, poultry, or vegetables. The flavor permeates, but because they are drained off, they add virtually no calories.

Regular mayonnaise has 11 grams of fat and 100 calories per tablespoon; light mayo has 5 grams fat and 50 calories; fat-free mayonnaise has 0 grams of fat and 10 calories. Whipped mayonnaise-type dressings have 7 grams of fat and 70 calories; light dressings have 3 grams of fat and 40 calories; nonfat varieties have 0 grams of fat and 15 calories per tablespoon.

Look at the sodium level listed on the Nutrition Facts panel, if sodium is restricted. Salad dressings vary widely in sodium content.

Xanthan gums and EDTA are safe additives frequently added to bottled dressings to thicken them, maintain their consistency, and lengthen their shelf life.

Alternatives for salad dressing that contain no fat include fruit, herb, and balsamic vinegars, salsas, and fresh lemon or lime juice with seasonings.

Cream and Cream Substitutes

Look For

➤ Reduced-fat or fat-free coffee creamers; half-and-half for selected uses.

➤ Reduced-fat, light, or fat-free sour cream or sour half-and-half.

➤ Ultrapasteurized products, which stay fresh longer in your refrigerator.

➤ Instant real whipped light cream in an aerosol can with only 1 to 2 grams of fat per tablespoon, or light or fat-free whipped toppings found in the freezer case.

Shoppers Should Know

Half-and-half is a blend of milk and cream. One ounce of half-and-half (about 2 tablespoons) has 40 calories and 3 grams of fat. Adding it as liquid cream to coffee can add considerable calories and fat if several cups of coffee are consumed daily. Try substituting whole milk, evaporated fat-free milk, or powdered fat-free milk to boost calcium intake.

Sour half-and-half, also called reduced-fat sour cream, contains about 45 calories and 3 to 4 grams of fat (2 to 3 grams of saturated fat) in a 2-tablespoon serving.

Real sour cream has 6 grams of fat per 2 tablespoons. Sour half-and-half can be substituted for most uses without much change in flavor.

Fat-free sour cream has 35 calories and no fat per 2-tablespoon serving.

Whipping cream contains about 45 calories and 5 grams of fat per tablespoon. One tablespoon yields about 3 tablespoons of whipped cream.

Cream in many recipes can be replaced with evaporated fat-free milk, whole milk, soy milk, or rice milk.

Liquid nondairy creamers contain no protein or calcium. They are often substituted for milk and cream in cooking or used to lighten coffee, but they do not provide the nutrients found in milk. They contain varying amounts of sugar and some are flavored.

Powdered coffee creamers may contain saturated fat and sugar. Check the Nutrition Facts panel and choose powdered creamer containing unsaturated fats if you use this product often. Powdered skim milk is a nutrient-rich substitution for powdered coffee creamer.

Regular chilled nondairy whipped topping has only 1.5 grams of fat per 2-tablespoon serving, but all the fat is saturated. Light and fat-free chilled whipped toppings are fairly low in fat but contain small amounts of hydrogenated vegetable oils and/or saturated coconut or palm kernel oil to maintain their consistency. Because these toppings have little or no measurable fat, however, they are reasonable choices.

Frozen Desserts

Look For
➤ Frozen low-fat and nonfat frozen yogurts—desserts that are sources of calcium and other key nutrients—in cartons,

bars, or individual cups. They are the most nutrient-rich frozen desserts.

➤ Frozen fruit or juice bars made with 100 percent fruit or juice are an excellent choice. Each bar counts as 1 serving from the Fruit Group.

➤ Low-fat ice cream with 3 grams of fat or less per serving. Fat-free varieties are also available.

➤ Low-fat frozen yogurt or ice cream bars coated with fruit sorbet.

➤ Fruit sorbets and fruit ices, which have no fat or cholesterol. Some provide vitamins C or A, depending on the type of fruit.

➤ Frozen fudge bars and pudding pops to provide extra calcium for less than 100 calories per serving.

➤ Ice milk and frozen low-fat milkshakes.

➤ Nondairy frozen desserts if lactose intolerant.

➤ Ice cream cups, sugar cones, or waffle cups to go with some frozen desserts.

Shoppers Should Know

Preportioned, single-serving items help curb the tendency to eat large portions.

Most frozen desserts fall within the Fats, Oils, and Sweets Group. Frozen yogurt, ice cream, and 100 percent juice bars are the exceptions.

Frozen yogurt is a good source of calcium and other nutrients provided by that food group. One cup of frozen yogurt counts as 1 serving from the Milk Group.

Some frozen yogurts have as much fat and sugar as light ice creams. Check the Nutrition Facts panel.

Sherbet is a milk-based frozen dessert with less fat than ice cream but more sugar.

Sorbets and granitas are sweetened frozen desserts usually made from fruits but sometimes with herbs. They contain no milk or cream and are fat-free and cholesterol-free.

Premium ice creams can have up to 26 grams of fat per 1/2-cup serving.

Some premium ice cream bars with chocolate coating have 22 grams of fat and 300 calories per bar. Reduced-calorie chocolate-covered ice cream bars are available.

Ice cream candy bars have 140 to 200 calories per bar and 7 to 13 grams of fat, though reduced-fat versions are available.

Sundae cones have 310 calories and 16 to 17 grams of fat. They have more calories and fat than a cone you fill with frozen yogurt or light ice cream.

Ice pops are colored, flavored water with added sugar.

Sugars, Syrups, Sweet Sauces, and Toppings

Look For

- ➤ Granulated white, confectioner's, and brown sugar and honey to use in moderation.
- ➤ Molasses. Its intense flavor and sweeteners allow you to use a small amount and, unlike other sweeteners, it provides some iron and calcium.
- ➤ Fruit syrups or real maple syrup—very intense flavors—to use in small amounts.
- ➤ Light or lite maple-flavored syrup—for reduced sugar and calories. Some have butter flavoring.
- ➤ Individual sugar packets or sugar cubes for portion control.
- ➤ Sugar substitutes if restricting sugar.
- ➤ Chocolate syrup, fruit, or low-fat or fat-free caramel, butterscotch, or fudge toppings for use over ice cream or frozen yogurt. All are low in fat but high in sugar—calories vary.

Shoppers Should Know

Brown sugar is sugar crystals with a bit of molasses. It has 50 calories per firmly packed tablespoon and tiny amounts of calcium, iron, phosphorus, and potassium—not enough to make a nutritional difference. Dark brown sugar has slightly more molasses. Light brown sugar uses the term "light" to describe the color and flavor. It is not lower in calories, carbohydrate, or other nutrients.

Confectioner's sugar is pulverized granulated sugar with a bit of anti-caking agent. It is used for frosting and sprinkling on foods. It has fewer calories per teaspoon than granulated sugar, and it now comes in lemon, strawberry, and chocolate flavors.

Corn syrup and high-fructose corn syrup are made by processing cornstarch to a thick sweetener containing several sugars. Frequently used in processed foods, corn syrup contains 60 calories and 15 grams of carbohydrate per tablespoon. Light corn syrup has a bit of added vanilla; dark corn syrup has a bit of caramel flavor.

Pure maple syrup is the sap of the sugar maple tree boiled down to a syrup. Less costly maple-flavored syrup (pancake syrup) is corn syrup with maple flavoring.

It is against the law to sell raw sugar in the United States because it is unrefined and contaminated with yeasts, molds, and soil.

When a food is labeled "no added sugar," it means that there is no added table sugar or other sweeteners like honey, corn syrup, or fruit juice concentrate. The product may contain sugars that occur naturally in that food.

Reduced-sugar foods contain at least 25 percent less sugar than the standard product.

Sugar-free means a food contains less than 1/2 gram of sugar per standard serving of that food. Other terms meaning the same thing are no sugar, sugarless, and without sugar.

Cinnamon toast made with cinnamon sugar is an economical low-fat alternative to sweet rolls. Mix your own cinnamon with sugar for an economy blend.

Most butter-flavored pancake syrups are fat-free.

Natural fruit syrups have 210 calories and more than 50 grams of sugar per 1/4-cup serving.

Chocolate and strawberry syrups and fat-free toppings both have about 80 to 130 calories per 2-tablespoon serving—about 25 grams of carbohydrate from sugar. Regular hot fudge topping has about 140 calories per 2-tablespoon serving with less sugar but 4 to 6 grams of fat.

Marshmallow cream topping provides about 90 calories per ounce, 23 grams of sugar, and no fat.

Frozen strawberries, raspberries, or peaches can be puréed to make a sweet sauce that is lower in sugar than syrups.

Never give honey to infants, small children, or people with

impaired immune systems. Honey can carry spores of botulism that are dangerous to those who have little resistance. Once swallowed, the spores can germinate, releasing toxins. Honey should not be put on pacifiers or in baby food, or added to tea given to individuals with impaired immune systems.

Jellies and Fruit Spreads

Look For

> ➤ Fruit preserves, marmalades, jams, and spreadable fruits.
> ➤ Fruit butters, such as apple, apricot, and peach butter.
> ➤ Reduced-sugar jams, jellies, and preserves, if limiting calories or carbohydrate.

Shoppers Should Know

Spreadable fruit is concentrated fruit with fruit juice used as sweetener instead of sugar. It has about the same amount of sugar and calories as jam or jelly—about 40 to 50 calories per tablespoon.

Contrary to what their name suggests, fruit butters contain no fat.

Fruit spreads and fruit butters on toast, English muffins, or bagels are a healthful, economical alternative to sweet rolls and doughnuts.

When using any fruit spread or fruit butter, omit or use less regular butter, margarine, or cream cheese to save on fat and calories.

Jellies are clear compounds of fruit juice, sugar, and pectin thickeners. Jams and preserves contain bits of fruit. Marmalades are made of citrus fruits and contain strands of the citrus rinds.

Reduced-sugar jellies, jams, and preserves have about half the sugar of regular ones, about 25 calories per tablespoon.

Artificially sweetened jellies, jams, and marmalades (including some light preserves) substitute artificial sweetener for sugar and contain a modified form of pectin that allows jelling to occur without sugar.

Combined Foods—Soups, Sauces, and Dips

Look For

➤ Vegetable, bean, chicken, seafood, and beef soups. Reduced-sodium or lower-sodium soups, if sodium is restricted.

➤ Split pea, bean, lentil, and barley soups. All are excellent sources of protein and fiber.

➤ Canned broth to be used to replace some or all of the fat in stir-frying.

➤ Low-fat dry soup mixes. They come in interesting flavors but are usually high in sodium.

➤ Vegetable broth, especially for vegetarians.

➤ Reduced-sodium sauces, if sodium is restricted.

➤ Canned or bottled gravies. Many are low-fat or fat-free and taste as good as homemade.

➤ Tomato-based pasta or pizza sauces with or without added vegetables or seasonings.

➤ Oriental sweet and sour sauces, char siu, and hoisin sauce. They are high in sugar but low in fat or fat-free.

➤ Salsas and picante sauces.

➤ Fruit sauces such as cranberry sauce and mango chutney.

➤ Bean dips made with black beans or pinto beans.

➤ Prepared onion and other low-fat dips made from nonfat dry milk. Two tablespoons contain about 30 calories and 8 percent of daily calcium needs.

➤ Low-fat, light, or fat-free chip and party dips.

➤ Light guacamole dip.

Shoppers Should Know

A standard serving of soup is 1 cup, about 8 1/2 ounces by weight.

Soups can be an excellent way to eat more vegetables, legumes, and grains.

Ready-to-eat hearty vegetable or chunky-style soups make a good entrée for a quick meal.

Condensed cream soups can be diluted with skim milk, water, or broth.

New England clam chowder (white) has more fat than

Manhattan-style clam chowder (red).

Cranberry sauce or chutney with pork or poultry is a tasty alternative to homemade gravy; mint sauce works well with lamb instead of gravy.

Prepared cheese, pesto, and clam sauces are likely to contain considerable fat. Read labels carefully. Canned white clam sauce for pasta has more than twice the fat of canned red clam sauce. Check the Nutrition Facts panel.

Alfredo sauce is made primarily of butter, eggs, and cheese. Stroganoff sauce contains sour cream. Both are high in fat and, usually, sodium.

Bottled creamy sauces for chicken have 8 to 10 grams of fat in 1/2 cup. Cacciatore and sweet and sour sauces for chicken have 2 or less grams of fat per 1/2 cup.

Guacamole is made from avocados, which are high in fat— but the fat is monounsaturated.

Regular sour cream dips and seasoned cream cheese spreads are high in fat.

Prepared cheese dips vary in fat content. Check the label.

Blend cottage cheese or reduced-fat cream cheese with shredded cheese and seasonings to make homemade cheese dip.

Prepared Entrées

Look For

➤ Frozen full meals with less than 400 calories, 15 grams of fat, and 800 milligrams of sodium. Among regular frozen dinners, sirloin, teriyaki chicken, roast chicken, sirloin tips, shrimp creole, sliced turkey, ham steak, and some pasta entrées are generally the lowest in fat. Short ribs, fried chicken, cheese-filled manicotti, macaroni and cheese, Mexican combos, and fish and chips are generally among the highest in fat.

➤ Frozen entrées with no more than 300 calories and 10 grams of fat per serving. Frozen entrées that usually meet these criteria include spaghetti or mostaccioli with meat sauce, sliced beef or turkey with gravy, chicken cacciatore, green pepper steak, sirloin tips, chicken or beef teriyaki, chicken chow mein, shrimp creole, and any entrée labeled light.

➤ Whitefish or other cooked fish balls in broth. Each piece has 7 grams of protein, 60 calories, and only 2 1/2 grams of fat. Kids, even toddlers, often like this gefilte fish and fish balls.

➤ Canned turkey chili with beans, labeled 99 percent fat-free. It has only 200 calories and is high in fiber.

➤ Canned chicken in broth.

Shoppers Should Know

Check the Nutrition Facts panel to help you make wise food choices. Frozen meals and frozen and canned entrées vary widely in both serving size and nutrient content.

It's wise to compare serving sizes. Some frozen dinners are only 8 ounces; others are 19 or more ounces.

Most frozen meals do not contain a full serving of vegetables.

One standard serving of frozen pizza is about 1 (5-ounce) slice; 2 slices have twice the nutrients stated.

Each small single-serving beef or chicken pot pie (8 ounces) has 18 to 24 grams of fat.

Breaded or batter-dipped fried frozen foods are usually high in fat, calories, and sodium.

Adding a fresh green salad, bread, and fat-free or low-fat milk enhances the nutritional value of meals based on frozen entrées.

Canned pasta entrées vary widely in calorie and fat content. Read the labels and compare. Generally, pastas with tomato sauces are lowest in fat and calories.

Many canned entrées, such as ravioli and chilis, have more than 1,000 milligrams of sodium per 1-cup serving. Read labels carefully if on a sodium-restricted diet.

Canned beef stew has about half the fat of canned corned beef hash (13 versus 25 grams).

Canned chili with beans has more fiber than canned chili without beans. But even vegetarian chili may not be low in fat; one brand has 20 grams of fat per cup.

If restricting sugar, sweet and sour sauces should be avoided. One brand of boil-in-bag sweet and sour chicken has 63 grams of sugar in a 10-ounce package. One sweet and sour chicken frozen dinner has 66 grams of sugar.

Baked Desserts

Look For

- ➤ Baked desserts that provide Nutrition Facts on the label so you can make informed choices.
- ➤ Angel food cake, lady fingers, gingerbread, sponge-cake dessert shells, baked meringue shells, or other plain or low-fat cakes and baked goods to top with fresh fruit.
- ➤ Unfrosted or lightly frosted cakes.
- ➤ Small cupcakes, sweet rolls, and other single-serving desserts.
- ➤ Fruit-filled crepes and tarts—they usually have a smaller amount of rich filling than pies.
- ➤ Pumpkin or sweet potato pie—rich in beta-carotene and fiber.

Shoppers Should Know

Calories and nutrients are based on the portion size listed on the label. You may choose a larger or smaller portion.

Much of the fat and calories in pies is in the crust. Tarts, cobblers, and meringue- or crumb-topped fruit desserts usually have less fat than double-crust pies.

Think twice about any dessert that has more than 10 grams of fat or more than 4 grams of saturated fat per portion. Enjoy a small serving.

Words such as "homestyle," "all butter," and "premium" usually translate to high-fat, high-calorie.

Many fresh baked goods don't have a Nutrition Facts panel. Look at the first few ingredients on the ingredient list as a clue to probable fat content.

Enjoy small portions of high-fat favorite desserts occasionally. Balance high-fat desserts with plenty of fruits, vegetables, and plain grains in the same day or the next day.

Deli Choices and Carry-Out Foods

Look For

- ➤ Steamed, grilled, or roasted vegetables.
- ➤ Lean sliced roasted beef, turkey breast, pork, or baked ham.

- Grilled chicken breasts; rotisserie chicken. (Remove skin before eating chicken.)
- Poached or grilled fish, shrimp, or scallops.
- Surimi (imitation crab, lobster, or shrimp), made from seasoned pressed fish.
- Grain salads, pilafs, couscous, and rice mixtures.
- Italian beef, barbecued beef, and meat balls in marinara sauce.
- Pastas with tomato-based sauces.
- Turkey or other lean meats or veggies in rolled flour tortillas or in pita pockets.
- Low-fat tuna, crabmeat, and chicken salads.
- Black bean and other bean salads.
- Beet, potato, carrot, or cucumber salads without lots of mayonnaise.
- Raw cut fruits and vegetables.
- Vegetable and pasta salads with vinegar-type dressings. Excess liquid can be drained, which can't be done with creamy dressings.
- Ratatouille and other mixtures of cooked vegetables.
- Salsas and fruit or vegetable relishes.
- Fresh mozzarella cheese balls and feta cheese in water.
- Reduced-fat cheeses in slices or wedges.

Shoppers Should Know

Virtually all prepared foods are time-savers but command premium prices.

It's smart to ask how foods are prepared and if nutrient information is available. Because prepared foods seldom carry nutrition labeling, it is hard to know which are the best choices. Many stores have nutrition or ingredient information available even if it is not displayed. Ask the deli manager for product information.

Egg rolls, potato pancakes, and vegetable pancakes are usually deep-fried.

If buying fried food, buy larger pieces (chicken breast versus wing, larger pieces of fish). The percentage of fried surface is less—so there are fewer calories in the same weight of that food.

Mousses and pâtés are prepared with lots of butter or cream.

Up and Down the Aisles

Most deli sausages are high in fat.

Order sandwiches on French or Italian bread, on whole-wheat bread or rolls, or in pita pockets. Croissants and focaccia add a lot of fat to sandwiches.

Some deli sandwiches, particularly large sub sandwiches, have 900 calories.

Portions of some single-serve items in delis are often very large. Realize that a 12-ounce stuffed potato is at least 2 servings, giant muffins about 3 servings, and over-stuffed sandwiches 2 servings each of meat and bread. Count servings from the Food Guide Pyramid and calories accordingly.

Beverages—Coffee, Tea, and Cocoa

Look For

➤ Plain or flavored coffee and teas.

➤ Coffee beverages (latte, cappuccino, etc.) made with skim milk.

➤ Decaffeinated coffees, decaffeinated teas, or herbal teas or grain-beverages, if you are sensitive to caffeine.

➤ Iced tea mixes, with or without sugar.

➤ Green tea. It contains protective substances that may boost the immune system and may help reduce the risk of gastrointestinal cancers.

Shoppers Should Know

Because they contain no nutrients, plain coffee and tea (unless sweetened) are not required to carry a Nutrition Facts panel.

Some instant, flavored coffees made from dry mixes contain about 50 calories and 2 grams of fat per cup. They also contain considerable amounts of sugar, unless sugar-free. Brewed coffees made from ground, flavored beans are calorie-, sugar-, and fat-free.

Dry mixes for flavored coffees sometimes contain coconut oil or hydrogenated oils.

Decaffeinated coffee is brewed from beans that are at least 97 percent caffeine-free.

Caffeine occurs naturally in coffee, tea, kola nuts, and chocolate. In moderation, it is a mild stimulant. Drip coffee contains about 130 milligrams of caffeine per 5-ounce cup; standard brewed coffee about 80 milligrams; instant coffee about 60 milligrams; and decaf about 3 milligrams. The amount of caffeine in tea depends on how long it is brewed. It ranges from 25 to 50 milligrams per 5-ounce cup. A 5-ounce cup of hot cocoa contains about 5 milligrams of caffeine.

Bottled cappuccino and other coffee-based beverages vary in nutrient values—read the Nutrition Facts panel.

Iced frosty cappuccino and similar drinks made from syrups may be promoted as fat-free. Some of them have about 250 calories per glass, all from sugar. Real cappuccino or latte poured over ice cubes has a fraction of the calories and sugar. Ask for fat-free milk in cappuccino and latte to boost calcium and for less fat.

Bottled iced teas and tea-based beverages come with and without sugar and in many flavors. Some iced teas have almost as many calories as soft drinks.

Bottled or canned prepared iced tea or instant tea from mix is far more expensive than tea made from tea bags, which can be prepared and chilled in advance.

Soft Drinks, Sports Drinks, Water, and Flavored Waters

Look For

➤ Plain, sparkling, and flavored mineral waters, club soda, plain seltzers, sugar-free tonic water, sugar-free fruit drink mixes, and diet soft drinks. All have no calories.
➤ Water, juice, or sports drinks to replace fluid during and after physical activity.
➤ Caffeine-free colas and soft drinks if caffeine must be restricted.
➤ Regular soft drinks if extra energy or weight gain is needed.

Shoppers Should Know

Sweetened sodas and sweetened, flavored mineral waters have 130 to 210 calories per 12-ounce serving, all from sugar.

Corn syrup and high-fructose syrup are sugars used in beverages and are equal in calories to regular sugar. Some fruit-flavored sparkling waters contain a surprisingly high amount of sugar from these syrups.

Products containing noncaloric sweeteners indicate the type of sweetener used on the label. Nutrasweet (aspartame) and Sunnet (acesulfame) are the most commonly used calorie-free sweeteners.

Colas and some other soft drinks contain caffeine. Ginger ale, root beer, and most fruit-flavored beverages are caffeine-free.

Tonic or quinine water contains 90 calories per 8 ounces; diet tonic is calorie-free.

Sports drinks are blends of water, sugar, sodium, and potassium, often with artificial color and/or added flavor. Some are carbonated, and some are artificially sweetened. Unless exercise is sustained for one hour or more and the weather is hot, regular water will maintain hydration.

Buy the size of carbonated beverage you will use at one serving time. Two-liter bottles cost less per serving but lose their carbonation once they are opened.

Beverages packed in "sports bottles" command premium prices.

Wine, Beer, and Liquor

Look For
> ➤ Wine, beer, liquor, and other beverages containing alcohol for adults who choose to enjoy them in moderation.
> ➤ Alcohol-free beer or wine.

Shoppers Should Know

The Dietary Guidelines say, "If you drink alcoholic beverages, do so in moderation." Moderate alcohol use is 1 serving per day of wine, beer, or liquor for women, 2 servings for men.

A standard serving is 5 ounces of dry white or red wine, 12 ounces of regular beer, or 1 1/2 ounces of liquor.

Alcohol-free wines and beers usually contain fewer calories than their alcohol-containing counterparts.

Alcohol is second to fat in calorie value. It provides 7 calories per gram but few or no nutrients.

Research shows that moderate drinking, particularly of wine, may increase lifespan, and may lower risk of heart disease in some individuals. In some studies, moderate use of alcohol is linked with higher HDL or "good" cholesterol levels. Higher HDL may protect against heart disease.

Small amounts of alcohol can enhance the enjoyment of meals and promote relaxation, and may reduce blood pressure slightly.

Eighty-proof distilled spirits, such as Scotch, bourbon, and gin, contain 100 calories per 1 1/2 ounces. Gin, rum, vodka, and whiskey that are 100 proof (50 percent alcohol by weight) provide about 125 calories per 1 1/2 ounce jigger.

Liqueurs, which are sweetened alcohol-containing beverages, contain 150 to 190 calories per 1 1/2 ounces.

Most dry red and white wines have about 100 calories per 5-ounce glass; sweet dessert wines contain 90 calories in only 2 ounces.

Regular beer contains about 150 calories per 12-ounce bottle or can; light beer has 100 calories per 12-ounce bottle or can.

Children and adolescents, pregnant women or those trying to conceive, and individuals who plan to drive or do activities requiring good motor skills (such as using power tools) should not drink any alcohol.

Alcohol creates multiple health risks in anyone who consumes it in excess. People who are sensitive to alcohol, or who can not control drinking should avoid it entirely.

Alcohol interferes with the effectiveness of many medications. Speak to your doctor about potential problems if you take medicine and drink alcohol. With many prescribed medications, alcohol should be avoided.

Cook with wine you would drink—or use leftover wine. Cooking wines have added salt, used as a preservative, that changes their flavor.

When cooking with wine, liquor, or liqueurs, some of the calories and alcohol are burned off if there is prolonged cooking or very high heat.

Seasonings and Condiments

Look For

➤ A variety of herbs and spices to season foods.

➤ Small amounts of less frequently used dried herbs and spices.

➤ Fresh herbs for maximum flavor and color.

➤ Cider, balsamic, wine, or other flavored vinegars.

➤ Garlic, shallots, gingerroot, horseradish, and other seasonings that add bold flavor without fat or salt.

➤ Mustard or flavored mustards, which are low-fat and low in sodium, as a seasoning or marinade.

➤ Salsas, barbecue, Worcestershire, chili, hot pepper, mint, seafood, and other low-fat or fat-free prepared sauces and seasonings.

➤ Asian sauces including teriyaki, reduced-sodium soy sauce, and tamari marinades and marinade mixes.

➤ Salt-free herb blends and light salt, reduced-sodium soy sauce, reduced-sodium chili sauce, and similar products if sodium is restricted.

➤ Fresh lemons, limes, oranges, and tangerines—for their zest and juice.

Shoppers Should Know

Liberal use of herbs, spices, and condiments allows reductions in fat and (sometimes) salt without loss of flavor.

Dried herbs and spices should be stored in a dry, cool, dark place. They lose flavor with age or when exposed to heat or light. Replace herbs and spices that have lost their fragrance or changed color.

Grate the zest from citrus fruits (lemons, limes, oranges, and tangerines) and use the zest and juice to season vegetables, grains, sauces, and marinades. Small amounts of citrus don't count as a serving from the fruit group but add lots of flavor to foods.

Generally, sources of sodium in the diet are one-third from sodium added to processed foods, one-third from salt (sodium chloride) added in cooking or at the table, and one-third from the sodium that occurs naturally in foods.

Kosher salt is a coarser grind than table salt. It has 480 milligrams of sodium per 1/4 teaspoon compared to 590 milligrams of sodium per 1/4 teaspoon in regular salt. Many chefs prefer kosher salt or sea salt for cooking.

Iodized salt contains a small amount of iodine, a trace mineral. Getting enough iodine used to be a problem for some people. Now, because food processing equipment is cleaned with solutions containing iodine, the tiny amounts needed are generally supplied by processed foods.

Ways to reduce or moderate intake of sodium or salt include: using salt sparingly, if at all, at the table; seeking lower-sodium choices by reading labels; and limiting intake of salted or high-sodium foods, such as most cheeses, frozen desserts, packaged mixes, canned soups, and salty condiments.

Baking Basics

Look For

➤ Pantry cooking basics including flour, baking powder, baking soda, yeast, flavor extracts, etc.

➤ Pure vanilla extract. It has a much better flavor and aroma than imitation vanilla flavor.

Shoppers Should Know

Cooking "from scratch" is generally less expensive and allows better control of the amount of fat, sugar, and salt used.

Flour is made from pulverized whole grains. All-purpose flour is wheat flour. The percentage of protein to starch varies among different types of flour. Bread flour is a bit higher in protein than all-purpose flour. Most all-purpose flour is presifted.

Most flour has been "bleached" with safe chemicals to make it lighter and whiter; unbleached all-purpose flour is available.

In enriched flour, a few of the vitamins and minerals lost in milling have been replaced and some folate is added. It is still lower in fiber than whole-wheat or other less-refined flours.

Baking powder is a mixture of starch, baking soda, and salts. It is used as a leavening agent in baking. Introduced in the mid-1800s as one of the first convenience foods, it is high in sodium (about 350 milligrams per teaspoon). Reduced-sodium varieties are available.

Baking soda, when activated by heat and liquid, particularly mild acids like buttermilk, releases carbon dioxide, which leavens batters and doughs. Baking soda provides 475 milligrams of sodium per 1/2 teaspoon. It is also an antacid. Its alkaline properties intensify the color of green vegetables but destroy their vitamin C content so it should not be used in vegetable preparation. Baking soda is an excellent, inexpensive household cleaner that neutralizes unpleasant odors.

All yeast is dated with a "use by" date. The "use by" date indicates how long a product will maintain optimal quality after you bring it home. Dry yeast products do not require refrigeration. Compressed fresh yeast is perishable and must be refrigerated until used.

Chapter Five

Keeping Food Safe

AMERICA IS BLESSED with one of the safest and most abundant food supplies in the world. Keeping food safe is a shared responsibility of farmers, manufacturers, distributors, retailers, the government, and, ultimately, consumers.

Eighty-four percent of shoppers say they are confident that supermarket food is safe—until there is a problem due to bacterial contamination, pesticide residues, or product tampering! But we shouldn't wait until there is a crisis to act. Most of the time, we could be more vigilant about protecting the food we buy and eat.

Safe Food for You and Your Family, another book in The American Dietetic Association's Nutrition Now Series, explores food safety issues such as the causes of foodborne illness; storing, handling, and cooking at home; eating away from home; and the effects of food additives, pesticides, biotechnology, and other food processes.

Here are some shopping tips to help you make safe food choices:

➤ Shop at clean and responsible stores and markets. Check display cases, shelves, and floors for cleanliness. Permanent facilities, like supermarkets, are more likely than farmstands to implement regular sanitation and pest control procedures. Stores with a high volume of sales are more likely to have greater turnover and fresher perishable foods.

➤ Buy food in excellent condition, such as fruit without cuts or bruises. Bruised or wilted produce has passed its peak or has been mishandled.

➤ Look for "sell-by" and "use-by" dates on perishable foods like milk, dairy products, bread, fresh meat, and cold cuts. The "sell-by" date is the last date that a food should be sold. Plan to use the item within a few days of that date. Choose items with the latest available "sell-by" date.

➤ The "use-by" date indicates how long a food will maintain its quality after you bring it home. If the "sell-by" or "use-by" date has passed, don't buy the product.

➤ Anything you buy frozen should be frozen solid and tightly sealed without evidence of previous thawing. Plain frozen vegetables (like corn or potatoes) should be separated, not frozen in a solid clump. Packages that are oddly shaped or with evidence of frozen liquids around the edges are likely to have been thawed and refrozen.

➤ Select frozen and refrigerated foods at the end of the shopping trip. Don't choose them first and then spend another 40 minutes shopping. They will thaw in your cart.

➤ Foods in bulk bins, salad bars, or self-serve bakery areas should be held at an appropriate temperature and protected by covers, lids, or plastic or glass sneeze guards. Each food should have its own separate scoop or utensil.

➤ Eggs, cheese, fresh meat, and poultry should be sold from refrigerated cases. Open egg cartons to ensure the eggs are clean and whole. Avoid cartons with any cracked eggs.

➤ Canned goods should be in labeled cans free of dents, leakage, rust, or bulges.

➤ Fresh fish and shellfish should be sold from cases that are well-chilled, with clean, fresh ice. Raw seafood in the case should be separated from cooked shrimp or other ready-to-eat shellfish.

➤ All fresh fruits and vegetables should be sold from clean display areas. Bagged salad greens and fresh-squeezed juices should be displayed in refrigerated cases to preserve quality. Some stores have water misters to preserve produce freshness. Potatoes, onions, and winter squash should be stored in cool, dry areas. They don't require refrigeration. Tomatoes and bananas should be neither sold from nor stored in refrigerated cases. Handle fresh fruits and vegetables gently. Place produce in your shopping cart and grocery bags where it won't get bruised. Damage and bruising promotes spoilage.

➤ Roadside stands and farmers' markets can supply wonderful, fresh produce but be extra careful to wash it well before eating it. Buy only pasteurized cider. Avoid buying shellfish, meat, poultry, or other highly perishable foods from temporary roadside stands or trucks. Buy fresh mushrooms only from known purveyors or stores. Wild mushrooms can look edible but be poisonous.

➤ Never buy any wrapped or packaged product in a poorly sealed container. In addition to a potential mess and spillage, there is the possibility of product tampering.

➤ If you see insects or rodents or any evidence of them, alert the store manager and/or city health department. Don't buy food at that store.

Use these hints to transport and store food immediately after purchasing it.

➤ Ask the bagger to pack all frozen and chilled items together to keep them cold longer. Put all raw meat, poultry, and seafood together to keep them from leaking on other foods. Take all refrigerated, chilled, and frozen foods home immediately and store them in the refrigerator or freezer as soon as possible.

➤ Be sure all food is bagged for transport in clean plastic or paper bags or in washed cloth or plastic carriers. Do not allow food to touch dirty car or truck storage areas or seats where pets have been carried.

➤ Store produce loosely wrapped or in covered containers. Fresh fruits and vegetables are safe as long as they are firm and there is no evidence of mold, a yeasty smell, or sliminess. Don't wash fruits and vegetables before storing them in the refrigerator (except salad greens you are cleaning and crisping). They will stay fresh and firm longer if washed just before eating.

➤ Read the safe handling instructions printed on some packages, particularly fresh meat and poultry. Some foods contain bacteria that can cause illness if the product is mishandled or cooked or stored improperly. The graphics tell you how to store and cook that food safely.

➤ Larger packages of fresh meat or poultry are often sold at a reduced price per pound. Divide large packages into meal-sized parcels. Wrap and seal them tightly in freezer bags, freezer paper, or plastic containers. Label packages with contents and date purchased. To maintain quality, repackage foods immediately after shopping when they are very fresh. Don't refrigerate food for several days before repackaging it for the freezer.

➤ Fresh meat and poultry covered with plastic film is not wrapped appropriately for freezer storage. Use freezer paper, foil, or plastic wrap to overwrap the original packaging material.

And don't forget to:

➤ Thoroughly rinse poultry and seafood in cold running water before cooking it. Scrub the shells of shellfish with a scrub brush. Use a separate cutting board for raw fish, poultry, meat, and seafood—one that is not used to cut produce and other foods you will eat raw. Don't let raw juices of poultry, meat, fish, or eggs touch other foods. Wash your hands before and after handling these foods. Also wash cutting boards, sinks, and utensils that have touched raw poultry, meat, and seafood with hot, soapy water and sanitize them after each use.

➤ Wash produce under cold, running water or in a colander to remove surface sand, dirt, insects, pesticides, and contaminants. Clean root and other firm vegetables and fruits with a vegetable brush or peel them. Use a chemical fruit and vegetable wash or a mild liquid soap to wash produce that may have been exposed to pesticides or bacteria.

➤ Discard any food that has evidence of mold or spoilage or that smells bad. The Department of Agriculture says, "If in doubt, throw it out." If you have just purchased it, return the food immediately for a refund.

➤ Check your refrigerator, freezer, and pantry and use existing stores of food first when planning menus. Periodically, clean out your pantry and refrigerator and discard foods that are very old (and of questionable quality and safety). Discard frozen foods with evidence of white, dry patches of freezer-burn or partial thawing.

Keeping food safe and maintaining a clean kitchen protect you and your family from potentially severe and sometimes recurring illness. Many people who have frequent gastrointestinal upsets or "flu" are victims of bacteria harbored in cutting boards, sponges, utensils, and refrigerators. Thorough cleaning with soapy water and a mild bleach solution should be a regular kitchen routine. The few minutes it takes is a good investment in protecting the health of everyone who eats in your home.

Index

cocktail sauce, 77
cocoa mixes, 62
cocoa, 101
coconut, 83
  dried shredded, 60
coffee creamers, 89, 90
coffee, 100–101
  and milk, 63
colas, 102
Colby cheese, 67
cold cuts, 77–78
collard greens, 45, 48, 49
collards, 45, 47
condiments, 104–105
cones, ice cream, 91, 92
confectioner's sugar, 92–93
constipation, and dietary fiber, 13
convenience foods, 27–28
cookies, 40
cooking fats, 86–87
cooking, and wine, 103
corn soufflés, frozen, 49
corn syrup, 15, 93
  and beverages, 101–102
corn, 45, 49
  creamed, canned, 50
  fresh, 44, 46
corned beef hash, canned, 97
Cornish game hens, 72
cornmeal, 37, 38
cottage cheese, 66
  creamed, 67
cottage cheese, dry curd, 67
coupons, 22–23
couscous, 37
  and carrot juice, 51–52
crab, 75
  imitation, 75
cracked wheat, 37
crackers, 39
  animal, 40
  graham, 40
cranberries, sweetened, 59
cranberry juice, 59
crayfish, 75, 76
cream cheese, 66
cream of rice, 37

cream of wheat, 37
cream substitutes, 89–90
cream, 63, 89–90
creamers, nondairy, 90
crepes, fruit-filled, 98
crispbreads, 39
crisps, 41
croissants, 33
  and deli sandwiches, 100
croutons, 33
crumpets, 31
crustaceans, 76
cucumbers, 45, 46
cupcakes, 40
custards, 68

daily value percentages, 14
dairy products, 61–68
  organic, 64
dandelion, 45, 48
dates, and young children, 60
deli foods, 26, 98–100
dental problems, 9
desserts
  baked, 98
  frozen, 90–92
diabetes, 8
  and chocolate milk, 63
diet, healthful, 8–10
Dietary Guidelines for Americans,
  8–9
dill, 46
dips, 95–96
dough, cookie, 40
doughnuts, 33, 40, 42
dressings, salad, 88–89
  and vegetables, 42
  homemade, 81
drink mixes, 59
duck, 72, 74

EDTA, and salad dressings, 89
egg bread, 33
egg rolls, 99
egg substitutes, 35, 80–81
eggnog, 61, 63
eggplant capanota, 50

fruit sauces, 95
fruit spreads, 94
fruit syrups, 93
fruit
  and food safety, 108, 109
  as snack, 55
  canned and bottled, 57–59
  dried, 54, 59–60
  fresh, 52–56
    selection of, 52–53
  frozen, 56–57
    vs. fresh, 57
  heavy vs. light syrup, 59
  irradiated, 56
  labels for, 11
  organic, 55–56
  washing of, 55
fudge topping, 92

game birds, 72–74
game meats, 69–72
garbanzos, 51
garlic bread, 33
garlic, 44, 104
  and allylic sulfides, 48
  bottled, 50
generic foods, 25
genestein, and soy, 80
Giardiniera, 50
ginger ale, 102
ginger, 44
gingerroot, 44, 104
gluten sensitivity, 34
gluten-free grains, 38
goat cheese, 66
goat, 70
goats milk, 61, 63
good source, definition of, 16–17
graham crackers, 40
grains, 37–39
  and carrot juice, 51–52
  gluten-free, 38
  quick-cooking, 38
granitas, 91
granola bars, 40
granola-type cereals, 37
grape leaves, stuffed, 50

grapefruit juice, 54
grapefruit, 53, 54
grapes
  and quercitin, 56
  freezing of, 57
  selection of, 53
gravies, 95
great Northern beans, 50, 51
greens
  canned, 50
  collard, 45
  salad, 44
grilling, 70
grits, 37
grocery shopping, 21–29
  and coupons, 22–23
  and rebate certificates, 22–23
  for variety, 22
  from home, 28
  money saving tips, 22–28
Gruyere cheese, 67
guacamole dip, 95
guacamole, 96
guavas, 54
guinea fowl, 72

half-and-half cream, 63, 89–90
ham, 69–72
  canned, 72
hash browns, frozen, 49
Havarti cheese, 67
health claims, and food labels,
  17–18
healthy, definition of, 17
heart disease, 8
  and alcohol, 103
  and antioxidants, 56
  and fiber, 13
  and omega-3 fatty acids, 75–76
  and soy, 79–80
herbs, 104–105
  fresh, 44, 46
herring, 75
high blood pressure, 8
high fiber, definition of, 17
high in, definition of, 17
hoisin sauce, 95

home replacement products, 27
honey, and children, 93–94
honeydew melons, 54
horseradish, 104
hot dogs, 77, 78
hummus, 79
hydrogenation, and peanut butter, 83
hypertension, 8

ice cream bars, 91–92
ice cream, 91
 homemade, 81
ice milk, 91
ice pops, 92
iced tea mixes, 100
ices, fruit, 91
indoles, 48
ingredient lists, 15–16
iodized, salt, 105
iron
 and dried fruits, 60
 and frozen vegetables, 49
 and fruit, 55
 and meat, 70
 and vegetables, 47
irradiation, and fruits, 56
Italian bread, 33

Jarlsberg cheese, 66
jellies, 94
jicama, 46
juice boxes, single-serve, 59
juice
 100 percent, 59
 calcium-fortified, 57
 canned and bottled, 57–59
 carrot, 51–52
 cider, 55
 fortified, 59
 fresh, 52–56
 fruit concentrate, 57
 tomato, and vitamin C, 51
 vegetable, 50

kale, 45, 47, 48, 49
kamut, 37

kasha, 37
kefir, 65
kidney beans, 51
 canned, 50
kiwi, 54
kohlrabi, 45
Kosher salt, 105
kosher symbols, 18

labeling laws, exceptions to, 11
labels, food, 11–19
 and deceptive practices, 19
 and health claims, 17–18
 and Nutrition Facts, 12–14
lactose intolerance, and frozen
 desserts, 91
lactose, and milk, 62
lady fingers, 40
lamb, 69–72
lard, 86
lasagna, 37
lavosh, 1, 39
lean meat, definition of, 17
leeks, 45
 and allylic sulfides, 48
legumes, 45, 78–80
 canned, 50
 and Food Guide Pyramid, 51
lemon juice, frozen vs. fresh, 57
lemons, 53
lentils, canned, 50
lettuce, 44, 46
 iceberg, 46
light foods, definition of, 17
lima beans, 45, 49, 51
 canned, 50
limes, 53
limonene, and citrus fruit, 56
liquor, 102–103
liverwurst, 78
lobster, 75, 76
lobster, imitation, 75
loquats, 54
lotus root, 45
low-calorie, definition of, 16
low-cholesterol, definition of, 16
low-sodium, definition of, 16

lox, 77
luncheon meats, 77–78
lycopene, 48

macaroni and cheese, 38
mackerel, 75
mangos, 53, 54
manicotti, 37
manufacturers, food, contacting, 16
maple syrup, 93
margarine, 84–86
   and pasta and grains, 38
marinades, 104
marmalades, 94
marshmallow cream topping, 93
matzo, 31, 39
mayonnaise, 88, 89
meat substitutes, 78–80
meat, 69–72
   and Food Guide Pyramid, 70
   and food safety, 109, 110
   cured, 72
   extra lean, definition of, 17
   game, 69–72
   grades of, 71
   labels for, 11
   lean, definition of, 17
   packaged, 77–78
   preparation of, 70–72
   selection of, 70–72
   serving sizes of, 70
medications, and alcohol, 103
melba toast, 39
melons, 54
   honeydew, 54
   ripening of, 55
   selection of, 53
meringue cookies, 40
meringues, uncooked, 81
milk, 61–64
   adjusting to lower fat content, 63
   and cereal, 37
   and Food Guide Pyramid, 62
   chocolate, 63
   condensed, 61

dry, 62, 63
evaporated, 63
fortified, 62
goats, 63
selection of, 62–64
millet bread, 34
millet, 37, 38
mint sauce, 104
mint, 46
miso, 78, 80
mix, trail, 41
mixes, baking, 35
molasses, 92
mollusks, 76, 76
monounsaturated fat, and nuts, 83
mousse, 68, 99
mozzarella cheese, 66
Muenster cheese, 66
muesli, 37
muffin mixes, 35
muffins, 31, 34
mushrooms, 44
mussels, 75, 76
mustard greens, 48, 49
mustard, 45, 104

National Shellfish Sanitation Program, 75
nectarines, 54
Neufchatel cheese, 66
neural tube birth defects, and folate, 18, 34
neurological conditions, and antioxidants, 56
niacin, and meat, 70
nondairy creamers, 90
noodles. See pasta
nut butters, 82–84
Nutrasweet, 102
nutrient content claims, 16–17
nutrients
   as expressed as percent of daily value, 14
   as listed on food label, 12–15
   permitted content claims, 16–17
Nutrition Facts label, 12–14

spirits, distilled, 103
sports drinks, 59, 101–102
sprays
    butter-flavored, 84, 86
    non-stick cooking, 86
spreads, 84–86
    fruit, 94
    sandwich, 88
sprouts, 44
    Brussels, 45
squab, 72
squash, winter, 43, 45, 46, 48, 49
squid, 76
starfruit, 54
steak tartare, 71
stew, beef, canned, 97
store brand foods, 25
strawberries, 53, 54
stroganoff sauce, 96
stroke, 8
stuffing mixes, 35
sucrose, 15
sugar alcohols, and tooth decay,
    18
sugar cones, 91
sugar, 8–9
    and daily value percentages, 15
    in cereal, 36
    raw, 93
    table, 15
sugar-free, definition of, 16
sugars, 92–94
sulfites
    and dried fruits, 60
    sensitivities to, 19
sulfur dioxide, and dried fruits, 60
Sunnet, 102
surimi, 75, 76
sushi, 77
sweet and sour sauce, 95
sweet potatoes, 45, 46, 48, 48
sweet rolls, 33, 40
sweet sauces, 92–94
sweeteners
    and beverages, 102
    artificial, and cereal, 37
Swiss chard, 45, 48

Swiss cheese, 66
syrups, 92–94

table sugar, 15
taco shells, 34
tahini, 82, 83
tangerines, 54
tapioca, 68
tarts, fruit-filled, 98
TBHQ, 37
tea, 100–101
teff, 37, 38
tempeh, 78, 79
teriyaki sauce, 104
terpenes, 48
    and oranges, 56
textured vegetable protein (TVP),
    80
tofu, 78, 79
    silken, 80
tomato juice, 59
    and vitamin C, 51
tomato-based sauces, 95
tomatoes, 43, 45
    and lycopene, 48
    canned, 50
    seasoned, 52
    storage of, 46
tonic water, 101, 102
tooth decay, sugar alcohols and, 18
toppings, 92–94
tortellini, 37
tortillas,
    corn, 34
    flour, 31
tostado shells, 34
trail mix, 41
triticale, 37
tropical oils, 88
trout, rainbow, 75
tuna, 75
    canned, 76
turkey, 72–74
    and safe preparation, 74
    self-basting, 73
turnip greens, 47, 48, 49
turnips, 45